Sweden

Aram Tofek

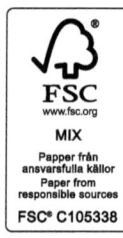

FSC
www.fsc.org
MIX
Papper från
ansvarsfulla källor
Paper from
responsible sources
FSC® C105338

Illustration: Aram Tofek

Förlag: BoD · Books on Demand, Stockholm, Sverige
Tryck: Libri Plureos GmbH, Hamburg, Tyskland

ISBN: 978-91-8057-558-4

Innehåll

Infromation around political circumstances

During most of the pandemic from 2020 up untill September 2022 the biggest politcial party in the goverment were Socialdemokraterna whoose party leader Stefan Löfven(So), now retired, were the prime minister. The other parties were Miljöpartiet, Centerpartiet and Liberalerna who left the government in July 2021. Vänsterpartiet supported the government, but were not officially in. The parties in the political opposition were Sverigdemokraterna, Moderaterna, Kristdemokraterna and Liberalerna from July 2021.

Shortenings

(So) – A politician active in Socialdemokraterna

(Mp) – A politician active in Miljöpartiet

(C) – A politician active in Centerpartiet

(L) – A politician active in Liberalerna

(V) – A politician active in Vänsterpartiet

(Sd) – A politician active in Sverigdemokraterna

(Mo) – A politician active in Moderaterna

(B) – A politician active in Bondeförbundet in the past

Explanations of autohorities and other things

The times of India, newspaper in India
Ekuriren, newspaper in Sweden
Aftonbladet, newspaper in Sweden
Dagens Nyheter, Newspaper in Sweden
Socialistinternationalen, Organisation of Socialist parties
UNWRA, United nations works for Palestinian refugees
UN, United nations works to maintaining international peace and security
Irish Oireachtas Commitee, Irish Parliament
WHO, World Health Organisation works to promote health internatioanlly
ECDC, Responds to infectious diseases in Europe
Skandinaviska Enskilda Banken, Bank in Sweden
MSB, Authority that works for the preparedness of Sweden
Arbetsmiljöverket, Authority for work enviroment in Sweden
Försäkringskassan, Gives money when people are off work due to sickness and other things
LO, The Union in Sweden
SIFO, Does surveys in media
SOS Alarm, Call center for Sweden
1177, A collection of information on healthcare
Socialstyrelsen, Authority who support Swedish healthcare
Folkhälsomyndigheten, Authority for public health
Coronakommisionen, Commision who reviews Sweden's handling of Corona
Smittskydd (Smittskydd Skåne), Works to reduce transmission of infection

1.1 Introduction

I can not say that the government wanted to kill people, however the naivity of the government and *Folkhälsomyndigheten* got the death toll for Covid-19 cases higher than necessary. The government were very passive during the pandemic and relied upon the expertise of *Folkhälsomyndigheten* and Anders Tegnell in particular.

The governemnts focus for the Corona strategy were protect the elderly, however since Sweden has a system where elderly are more prone to be at elderly care homes than on their own or with their adult children it is crucial that the elderly care homes are functioning. This is unfortunately not the case.

The law of Jante makes Sweden want to stand out from othe countries politically, but at the same time makes Swedes not want to stand out from eachother. The leading creators of the corona strategy for Sweden has therefore made the strategy unique from other coutreis´ strategies. This is to boost the Sweden image that they are obssessing over to keep great.

During World War II people that did not fit the ideal of the Nais were killed. Specifically the Jews. During corona, the elderly were targeted due to the government wanting to save money on pensions.

The plan of killing the elderly has been acheived through direct and indirect measures and came fro the idea of *Folkhemmet*. The bureaucracy of Sweden were used during World War II as well as during Corona to target a specific group. For corona it was the elderly.

1.2 Jantelagen

The following rules are the rules of Jante:

- You shall not think you are something
- You shall not think you are as good as us
- You shall not think you are more clever than us
- You shall not imagine you are better than us
- You shall not believe you are more than us
- You shall not believe you are more beautiful than us
- You shall not believe that you are fit for something
- You shall not laugh at us
- You shall not think someone cares about you
- You shall not think you can teach us something[1]

The law of Jante is an unwritten law in Sweden that is used quite frequently politically and it has shown in how Sweden has handled the corona pandemic.

1.3 Folkhemmet

The thought process behind *Folkhemmet* meaning the Swedish welfare is that in the words of Per Albin Hansson was a meaningful step forward towards "cleansing" the Swedes and "rinse" them from reproduction of inheritance that leads to undesirable individuals in future generations.[2] During the Covid-19 pandemic the focus has been on protecting the elderly, however that is exactly what the governmennt has not done. They have instead lowered the chances for their survival.

2.1 Folkhemmet erstwhile

Sweden sterilized about 62 000 Swedes based upon racial biology between the years 1934 to 1974.[2] 70 percent of the people that was sterilized was women[3]. The sterilisation process was natural to the Swedes and did not raise questions.[4] The sterilisations were part of the welfare, the so called *folkhemmet*; innocent people that were considered inferior in different ways were sterilised.[3]

The social democrat Gunnar Myrdal(So) active in *Socialdemokraterna* from 1934 and advocated for forced sterilisation of "incompetent humans". It stemmed from his idea to create a healthy, strong and productive population. He was inspired by Rudolf Kjellén(So).[5 s.225] Kjellén(So) is the social democrat who is responsible for Sweden´s corporate state system.[5 s.221] He wanted big welfare programs and a state with a progressive force built on people´s insitutions.[5 s.222] Myrdal(So) contributed to the race politics that the Americans used and was an editor for the study "An American Dilemma: The Negro Problem and Modern Democracy" that came out in 1944. In his study he concluded that the animosity between whites and blacks gave birth to each other.[5 s.226]

Axel Hägerström was a philosopher, socialist, and theologist. His ideas about morals came from vaue nihilism. Value nihilism rejects morals and ethics and says that rejects morals and ethics and says that you could not confirm ethics in practice, rather ethics is predetermined by the people in power. He became the high priest in the church of the Social democrats.[5 p.320] It was value nihilism in combination with Kjellénic principles gave the social democrats the right to sterilise women.[5 s.321]

The race biology institute opened in 1921 because the Swedish plans for it was not affected by World War I unlike other countries. The race biology institute was in Uppsala was initiated by Alfred Petrén(So) from *Socialdemokraterna* and Nils Wholins(B) from *Bondeförbundet* run by Herman Lundborg(B). *Bondeförundet* was the Swedish political party Centerpartiet of that time. The institute was voted for by the entire parliament. Petrén and Wholin later became advocates for the productivity of forced sterilisations.[5 s.233]

Sterilization was described as a "Human solution" to improve the circumstances for the misfits while reducing the social and economic burden they placed on society.[4] It was part of the Swedish welfare which was called *folkhemmet*. The idea was that Sweden was a home for the Swedish citizens and that nobody would starve or die.[6] Swedish politicians defended the sterilisation programs as they thought it was a good thing to to limit the size of families as that would limit the cost for the welfare state.[3] There was a broad consensus between medical communities and political parties that the sterilization programme would be a scientific and modern way to make society better.[4] The Peasant party and the Social democrats called on to prevent degradation of the Swedish nation and the researchers at the racial biology institute suggested that the degradation of the Swedish nation came from the violation of its purity.[4]

The law that was passed in 1934 approved sterilization without consent on people who suffered from insanity, feeblemindedness, other mental disorders, did not have good learning abilities, people who were considered "non-Aryans" and who was deemed to have defective genetic traits according to Von Hofsten referenced in Shaw & Kurbegovic.[7,8] It was the health or social welfare authorities that declared if people were eligible for sterilisation. An example of someone that was sterilised due to bad learning

7

abilities was a 13-year-old girl that was sterilised because she did not learn catechism and someone else was sterilized for not having good eyesight while not having access to glasses. Later the definition for inferiority expanded and started to include asociality and dangerous criminals and men with unusual or excessive sexual desires[8] and when you could change your sex, people who went through sex changes had to be sterilised, if they did not conform the sex change procedure be cancelled.[9] The sterilisation legislation was liberalised in 1964 and in 1976 the last sterilisation of the mentally disabled took place,[8] however the sterilisation of transgenders went on until 2013.[9] Couples who were considered to be inferior parents were sterilized and so were their children when they became teenagers.[3]

Sweden´s establishemnet of a race biology institute helped bring the ideology of Nazi Germany[3]. The origin of the sterilization program is in the study of eugenics which advocates for human engineering to create a superior race which is the core of the ideology Nazism.[3] The Law for the Prevention of Progeny with Hereditary Diseases came based upon recommendations of scientists involved in eugenics in July 1933 in

Germany and Adolf Hitler signed it and the following year a similar law was passed in Sweden[4]. Heinrich Himmler trusted the Swedish doctor Herman Lundborg to make sure that his SS-soldiers and their wives were "racially pure" and had the right skull shape.[5 p.234]

2.2 *Folkhemmet* currently

The politicians are trying to systemize the healthcare in a factory type model so that they can measure everything.[10 35:30-36:00] The politicians gives the healthcare workers more guidelines, administration and less freedom to analyse the patient and treat them accordingly. The politicians have done it so that the healthcare workers follows directions. If the directions are not helping, the healthcare workers has another set of directions that they have to follow.[10 34:17-34:59] When the politicians change the way of treatment, the healthcare workers must follow the new guidelines and it takes a lot of mental energy to take the new information in. These guidelines are sent out to all kinds of specialties in healthcare.[10 36:30-37:10] It has led to old people get palliative care right away when they have Covid-19 before seeing a doctor. When they are written for palliative care then they are excluded from hospital care, oxygen, fluids, food and other medication such as medicine that dissolves blood clots.[10] [27:10-28-32] When Jon Tallinger came to Denmark, he asked his boss about Denmark´s healthcare directions and the boss said that there were none.[10] [39:59-40:34]

The region of Stockholm is the richest region in Sweden, however there is errors with the hospital Södersjukhuset; elderly patients were left without food and care for 24 hours and they were waiting times of 24 hours as well.[11] In conjunction with this, they need to save 80 million Swedish crowns in 2021[12] and an additional 200 million for 2022 and 2023 for staff costs.[13] The hospital of Danderyd and Södertälje has economic problems as well. The hospital of Södertälje will have to do cost reductions that corresponds to 150 full time workers Socialdemokraterna made a motion to give the hospitals 312 million Swedish crowns in 2020, but it was not voted through. Today the hospitals would need 350 million and GPs and health centers needs 500 million. The amount of healthcare places has remained still[11] and is around 222 per 10 000.[14] The rise of corona cases in December 2020 resulted in Sweden reaching 99% of its intensive care unit capacity.[15] The normal number of operations that are done in a day in all hospitals in Sweden is 1010. During the pandemic, that has been reduced by 232 a day for 2020 respective 196 a day for 2021. The amount misssed operation for 2020 is 84 962 and for 2021 71 460 that is 156 422 operations in total for both years. The amount of time that it takes to recoup the operations is about 15 500 days meaning 42,5 years given that they do ten more operations a day.[16] The amount of time that someone had to wait for operation against colon and rectal cancer was nine to ten weeks in 2017. Bowel cancer specialists was not happy about it and alarmed politicians and managers, however in the following year the operation cue times became 15 to 17 weeks. The result was that the patients that were waiting became non-curable.[17] Sweden has the lowest amount of intensive care places per capita in Europe; it is precisely five per 100 000 which means a total of about 500.[18]

In the 1980s Sweden started to build military healthcare as a part of the total national defence. It had 125 000 emergency places, 88 000 extra beds and schools that could be transformed into care annexes within five days. Sweden had 50 extra hospitals, 35 field hospitals and 15 marine hospitals. Every field hospital had six operation rooms and an intensive care department each with 18 respirators. All of this was discontinued in the 1990s. It was discontinued by governments from both the political right and the political left.[19] During the Covid-19 pandemic Sweden set up two field hospitals; one in Göteborg with a capacity of 20 and one in Stockholm with the capacity of 30. The other field hospitals were given away or discarded during the early 2000s. All field hospitals would have not been useful today because of the high costs for upgrades to modern standards.[14]

The hospital of Salhgrenska was supposed to be free from corona patients[20] and therefore Sahlgrenska decided to use a field hospital for the corona patients; thus some intensive care places at the hospital became empty.[21] In the field hospital in Göteborg doctors said that there is no water or drains, the patients were located closer to each other than in normal departments. The ventilations are bad and the respirators are outdated.[22] Every corona patient is not taken care of in the field hospital, the most seriously ill are taken care of inside the hospital.[23] A doctor said that the hospital care in the field hospital is not the best intensive care that could be given.[24] The operations manager

Henrik Sundman said that the hospital care in the field hospital is of the same quality as in the hospital and that he sees it develop further.[25] After critique of the field hospital, it was decided that the corona patients would be taken care of inside the hospital.[26]

The emergency call center in Stockholm, Skåne, Västra Götaland and Halland had more calls coming in than they could normally handle on the 8th of January 2005. Halland had as many calls as they would normally receive during a day in an hour. Skåne has norally 200 calls to answer, however they received 1500. The emergency calls in Göteborg doubled from 1500 to 3000. People usually wait about eight seconds, but on that day the callers waited so long that they let 50 to 60 signals pass by. Callers who ended the call to call again would end up last in the queue and even though someone end the call, it still takes up a place in the queue. It is only Stockholm who has voice mails that confirms that the call has been answered and gives the caller its queue placement since the queue times are normally eight.[27] During more recent times, it has not become any better. The region of Västra Götland decided for nurses to receive emergencty calls during the Spring of

2019, however it failed; Nurses did not have the time to answer the calls, and it has costed more than expected. The emergency call center would still be receiving calls, however only after 30 seconds if the nurses would not answer. When the political parties voted to remove or maintain the operation; they voted to maintain it.[28] About 30 alarm operators quit their job during Autumn 2021. The alarm operators can not take breaks or eat lunch and they often work extra which leads to sleep problems and stress. The workload can affect the operator to make mistakes in calls. A starnger who called for a boy who started choking had to wait three minutes. By the time that she got the call back the parnets of the boy had started driving to seek help. The calls has risen yearly, corona is not the only cause for the higher amounts of calls.[29] The calls to *SOS Alarm* had increased to 14 000 calls per day in the summer of 2021 from 9 000 normally, it is a ten percent increase from the previous summer. Two reasons for the increase of callls was the pandemic and people on vacations within the country encounters crimes and accidents. There has also been calls due to people worrying about corona. Those kinds of calls is not what 112 calls are for it is rather 1177 that deals with those sorts of problems. Another type of wrong call is people reporting the smell of smoke when they are too far from the fire. About a third of the calls are done wrongly.[30]

A woman had breathing difficulties and her daughter called an ambulance; the case was rated a prio two meaning it is acute, but not fatal, however the ambulance went to a prio one and the woman did not receive the planned ambulance. The daughter knew of it only after calling back after 40 minutes. The woman received an ambulance 20 minutes after the second call.[31] A man in Norrbotten had been driven to the emergency room and was sent home later. At home he had a nose bleeding and called for an ambulance. He was placed in a virtual waiting room. People are set in the vrtual waiting room when there is no ambulance or when they are low priority.[32] A person fell in his home and received immense backpain and he was not able to stand up. An ambulance was called and they helped him onto his couch. They declared it was not needed for him to be sent to the hospital and left. The person fell forwards later that night and received a nose bleed. The same ambulance came and they helped him into the car of his partner because they thought he did not need to be sent In the ambulance. He on the other hand had too much pain for it to work. During the night a new ambulance was called and he was sent to hospital with it. They ascertained he had a nose bleed, bleed in the head and a broken back.[33] A woman with a suspected blood clot was denied an ambulance. The emergency calll center denied an ambulance for her because she did not have a car herself and it was not seen as acute. Five hours later the son of the woman calls again and gets denined. In the third call a taxi driver said he was going to drive her since there was no ambulnaces and in the last call the ambulance came, but it was to late and the woman died.[34] The time for response for first priority cases increased by 66 percent between 2010 and 2015. The ambulances are more than they were ten years prior, however the amount of cases increased by 20 percent. In Munkfors it takes about 24 minutes to receive an ambulance during life threatening circumstances. In rural areas the roads makes the time for transport to be at least as long as the waiting time for an ambulance; they therefore have other treatment strategies or drugs in rural areas.[35] An ambulance was not sent to a woman which was suspected to have corona because an ambulance staff member refused and had an eight months old baby at home which was her excuse.[3] A customer at a pharmacy fell sick with headache, neck pain and vomiting. They called for an ambulance and after two hours they had to call again because it did not appear. It was not planned to be an ambulance for the customer because the ambulance unit denied the case. The call operator was allotted to the emergency department because the person fell ill on the hospital premises. When the emergency departement was called by the operator, they denied the case aswell and directed the operator to the ambulance unit. The operator had to call back and forth.[37] In two different cases the ambulance staff personell received the wrong number for the doctor. The staff had to call a doctor in the first case due to the person being on alcohol and drugs. In the second case, the person hallucinated. Both refused to travel in the ambulance.[38] An ambulance unit drove a person to x-ray him due to a bicykle accident. The unit were supposed to wait for the x-ray result and drive him to Hudiksvall if needed, however the ambulance unit decided to eat their lunch instead. An ambulance unit from Hudiksvall came and were frustrated that they were incapable of ease his pain.[39] An ambulance unit changed its staff mid a priority one mission during two instances. Tone of them was moved to another ambulance unit and the two others were warned.[40] A patient with hernia of the carotid artery, unmeasurable blood pressure and a spleen injury was driven to the hospital. The ambulance staff said that they had warned the hospital, however the hospital did not agree and therefore there were no doctor or room ready for the patient.[41] On a single week the amount of missions increased by 15 percent. During the week there was 5 586 missions in total. The increase was due to covid-19, RS-virus, influenza and slip injuries. The staff did not have time for lunch and worked overtime often.[42] From the middle of June the ambulance of Vimmerby would only go on priority one alarms due to lack of resources. During 2021 less than 80 percent of priority one cases came to the patient in less than 20 minutes.[43] From a survey, it was ascertained that the wait times for ambulance are so long that if 10 000 Swedes received cardiac arrest every year roughly 600 would survive.[44] A man pulled his knee out of joint and he had to wait for three hours for an ambulance. The first car that was supposed to take the man, had another priority and therefore took the new mission. The ambulance staff provided him with pain reliever and drove him to the hospital.[45] An elderly man with cerebral haemorrhage was not driven to the hospital bevcause the ambulance staff made an assessment that he did not need to go to the hospital. The man lost his consciousness later that night and he later died.[46]

During 2015 about 163 000 people migrated to Sweden and they shall be offered a health checkup to evaluate their need for healthcare and to discover upcoming diseases that falls under the infection control law. In 2014 it was about 36 000 migrants who went through a health checkup and in 2015 the proportion of migrants that went through a health checkup was 38%, 64 000 migrants in total. The reason for the low amount of health checkups for migrants are that there is too much need for healthcare and specialized psychiatric care and trauma care in relation to its capacities.[47] From the graph over tuberculosis cases in Sweden comparing people born in Sweden and outside of Sweden published by *Folkhälsomyndigheten* the amount of cases were the same between the groups in 1992. Thence the group born outside of Sweden became bigger with 2015 having the most amount of foreign born cases.[48] After Somalian families was concerned about data indicative of Somalians being more likely to have autism. Somalian families stopped to vaccinate their children against measles, mumps and rubella.[49] The skepticism within Somalian families towards vaccines causing autismled to 30 percent of the citizens of Rinkeby and Tensta not taking the vaccines against measles.[50]

The amount of MRSA and ESBL cases increased during the first half of the 2010s to the point where it was considered a societal infection. ESBL cases had almost been double the cases of MRSA. A lot of cases has been among migrants from contries with less control and less restriction over antibiotic use. Half of the cases in Gotland were among migrants. The cases of MRSA doubled from 2015 to 2016 because of the 1 000 people who migrated in 2015.[51] MRSA has increased steadily since 2000.[52] MRSA are especially contagious in healthcare environments. During the period between 2008-2011 eight wound cares has had a total of 21 cases of MRSA.[53] Earlier MRSA was exclusively contagious within healthcare environments, however in 2017 half of all who tested positive for MRSA had been tested from ulcers or abscesses.[54] A lot of people who tested positive for MRSA migrated from countries with high MRSA incidence.[55] From 2005 to 2015 the amount of MRSA cases trippled from about 1 000 to 3 000. Tourism and migration are the reasons for the increase. The amount of MRSA cases in Syria has increased during the 2010s.[56] There has been lack of hygiene within the healthcare.[57] The ministry of social affairs does not include any preventive measures against antibiotics resistance that relates to immigration.[58 s. 8-9] While the amount of persons that contracted MRSA in hospitals halcved from 2006 to 2011, the amount of MRSA cases increased with 19 percent from 2010 to 2011. Only seven percent of cases had contracted MRSA in hospitals. ESBL cases increased in 2011 to.[59] From 2000 to 2003 the proportion of MRSA cases that was contracted abroad was 25 percent.[60] Anders Tegnell says that the increase of MRSA is because of trips and migration. Migrants can have injuries and wounds that are infected. They also say that MRSA cases increases because the testing of it has increased as if it is not obvious.[61]

The time you have to wait for a dental visit is six years in Skoghall.[62] The university hospital of Linköping is one of five hospitals in Sweden that does treatments for tumours of the esophagus and stomach and before they received patients from other regions, they already had long operation ques for those surgeries.[63] Patients with pancreas cancer can wait up to a maximum of four weeks if they want to become healthy, however in Lund the queue time for an operation can become eight weeks.[64] Out of the 35 analysed European countries Sweden, Serbia and Latvia are at shared last place when it comes to queue times for public care and Sweden is the second to last place in front of Portugal when it comes to queue times to see a family doctor. According to the same report Sweden, Malta and Bulgaria are the only countries that has not introduced healthcare laws based on patients' rights.[65] Sweden has the least amount of healthcare beds in Europe.[66] The cancer that you have to wait the longest for is prostate cancer, on average men have to wait 131 days for the operation. It is the most common cancer in Sweden while it has the longest queue time and kills the mst amount of people. There is a big difference between the regions; in Blekinge, the region with the lowest queue time, you have to wait on average for 81 days and in Västerbotten, the region with the lowest queue time, you have to wait on average for 260 days. The aim is that you should not wait for longer than 60 days meaning none of the regions meats the goal.[67]

An example of how the healthcare queue has increased is that in December 2014 there were 15 584 people waiting longer than 90 days for care and in December 2017 there were 33 402 people waiting longer than 90 days for care. In Sweden there is a statuatory care guarantee which says that one does only need to wait at most 90 days to receive a first meeting and wait another 90 days for the treatment. The increase between December 2014 and December 2017 which was the period where *Vänsterpartiet*, *Miljöpartiet*, and *Socialdemokraterna* reigned is about a 114 percent increase.[68]

Due to corona increasing the amount of patients at hospitals and the low amount of staff, cancer patients´ operations were cancelled during summer 2021.[69] Operations were cancelled in the region of Norrbotten because the region decided to ban hiring operating nurses. The new rule and the lack of healthcare places left hospitals with two choices; sending patients to other parts of the country or wait half a year for the operation. There is already about 200 patients who are sent to other hospitals elsewhere in the country. Every single patient who are sent elsewhere costs about 10 000 to 30 000. Some patients such as patients who needs prostate planning will have to go around with catheters.[70] Patients with pancreas cancer in Lund has been sent to Stockholm, Uppsala, Göteborg and Germany. In some cases the cancer has grown so much that the tumour is too big to operate away. During 2018 and 2019 the consultant Tingstedt reported six cases where patients cancer had gone too far before they received an operation time. Lack of hospital beds and operation times are inter alia due to lack of qualified personnel, it is hard to find and keep staff and staff taking sick leaves.[64] A patient with a heart diseas ecame in to the hospital of Kristianstad. He had breathing problems, however due to a lack of hospital beds, he were left untill the next day and died. When there is no beds left patients are left in corridors, shower rooms, staff rooms or at the wrong departement.[66] Bowel cancer specialist alarmed April 2017 that the queue time for a bowel cancer treatmnet was up to nine to ten weeks long. Up untill January 2019 the queue times increased to 15 to 17 weeks. According to *Socialstyrelsen*, patients should not have to wait longer than four weeks. The treatment should start within that timeframe. The surgeons wrote a letter to politcians stating that some patients wait so long that they become untreatable.[17] About 10 000 operations in Stockholm was cancelled in 2016 . Twelve patients with liver cancer were not able to be treated within the recommended timframe of 36 days at Karolisnska universitetssjukhuset. It was due to staff and care place shortage. The hospital of Danderyd offered to take care of some operations, however Karolisnska universitetssjukhuset is a solo contractor assignments which means that they take care of the current operations.[71] In 2019 six cancer patients had to be sent to Germany for their operation. Patients have also been sent to Nordic countries. The patients had cancer in their liver, bile ducts and pancreas. The Skånes universitetsjukhus sent a total of 56 patients in 2019, just five years prior, they sent none abroad.[72] A man with aggressive pancreatic cancer had to wait for two and a half months for the treatment, however half of the hospitals in Jämtland, two out of four, had a shortage of nurses; he decided to follow an advice he was given and had the operation in Germany.[73]

From an international perspective Sweden has a high proportion on doctors in relation to the population,[74] however they do not spent most of their time on their patients. A third of the doctors´ working hours goes towards their patients, a third to administrative work related to their patients and the last part of their work hours towards administrative work not related to their patients. It is the patient data act that determines what doctors should document which is too demanding. Medical secretaries has the education to ease the doctors´ administrative work burden. The County Council Administration initiates a lot of projects such as patient safety project or quality assurance that produces a lot of administration work for doctors where the administration becomes more than the actual act in itself.[75] A study was made with the goal of studying how all proffesions within eleven health centers spent their time; it showed that the average for all proffesions is that 30 percent of the time is spent on direct meetings with patients, 35 percent are spent on indirect patient time such as invitations, referrals and more and the rest 35 percent of the time goes towards meetings and workplace meetings. Nurses only sees patints for 20 percent of their work time.[76] Some things doctors do that takes their time from other things are bookings of trips, cleaning lunch roooms, and difficult and slow IT-systems.[74]

In 2005 4 000 patients died unnecessarily due to wrong information, accidents and error in managing patents. A common cause is that the lack of hygiene and routines leading to patients getting wound infections. There is also poor management when patients change their care giver due to the information exchange. There is also huge mistakes such as doctors confusing medicines, blood bags, operating on the wrong leg, starting the wrong treatment, reacting too late to symptoms or simply misdiagnosing.[77] In 2019 about 110 000 people are affected by injuries being in hospital, about 1 400 people die from them and 39 percent of the injuries can be avoided. Care-related infections, failure of vital functions, drugs and injuries due to surgical procedures are the most likely causes of care-related death. Surgical damages are the most common for care-related injuries that requires immediate life saving efforts or that gives permanent injuries. A reason for care related injuries are lack of competence because of lack of nurses and patients being in the wrong departemnet. Abour four percent of adult patients are moved; the care related injuries are 60 percent more for the moved patients and death is two times as common.[78] A patient was going to be revived, however other patinets was in the way of the life saving equipment due to them being take care of there since there was not enough hospital beds.[79]

A man came into the amergency departement with fever and pain. The staff did not prioritise him highly and there was not enough healthcare places; he died after ten hours due to blood poisoning because of meningitis.[80]

In 2015 it was believed that the migration would give Sweden a super economy, Sweden would receive a GDP growth of 4 to 5 percent and that Sweden would be the richest country in Europe three to four years later.[81] The migrants were seen as an economic investemnet. Instead the welfare suffered because the municipalities prioritised migration over the welfare. 180 out of 290 municipalities had to save money on health and social care before 2020. 209 municipalities had shortfalls within the elderly care. 60 percent of municipalities had to close schools.[82] The municipality of Gävle alarmed that they needed more money to maintain the quality of the welfare. The reason for it is that the municipality has increased by 1 000 people per year due to the increase of births and migration.[83]

The municipality investments went up to 193 billion in 2020 an increase of 9 billion in comaprison to 2019 and the loan debt increased to 726 billion in 2020 from the 659 billion loan debt of 2019. 63 municipalities decreased their loan debt, three municiaplities did not change their loan debt, however the rest 224 municipalities increased their loan debt. It is things such as an increasing population and the increase of young and old people that increases the demand of welfare as well as housing and real estate that needs renovations that costs money for municipalities.[84] For 2020 61 municipalities increased their taxes due to them predicting high migration. The rest of the municiaplities will instead save money on schools, elderly care and social services.[85]

The percentage of municipalities that will save money in each field. 214 out of 290 municipalities answered in the poll. 43% of munisipalities will save in other fields. How they will save is not specified.[86]

The municipality of Filipstad was about to crash in 2019 due to the high cost of immigration. The social benefits has multiplied and livelihood support has increased. The municipality received 6 to 7 billion from the sate, but needed about 100 million.[87] One of the expenses that migration has brought is municipalities giving migrants free driving lesson.[88] The high amount of migrants in Uppsala has led to higher costs. In 2015 the costs for contributions to migrants were 276 million sek, in 2018 the cost was 376 million sek and in 2019 it became 402 million sek.[89] Östra Göinge is a municipality that has increased its population through migrationn and they have experienced problems with not being able to finance the welfare because the migrants have not been able to get employed and the result will instead be that the subsistence allowance will get raised.[90]

A woman had metastasis in her lungs and liver from her colon cancer. She had been having chemotherapy and her doctor had told her that she only has two more years to live, however she decided to go to Germany for a hyperthermia treatment and it worked quite well. Normally you receive economic compenstaion for healthcare abroad; she did not receive the full amount 120 000 sek, she only received 3 000 sek because hyperthermia is not scientifically proven as a method against colon cancer.[91] A boy was misdiagnosed two times. At first the healthcare gave him paracetamol because of his headache when he was nine years. He was later diagnosed with migraine, however at last it was discovered that he had a brain tumour and hydrocephalus.[92] A girl suffered from a headache and her family seeked healtcare; she was sent home. After half a year the girl came back because she suffered from vomiting and visual disturbances also. They diagnosed her with tension headache with elements of migraine. The family was alloted to the emergency medical care, however the doctor did not think it was necessary. The girl became worse with her weight loss and problems and a squinting eye. Later it was discovered that the girl had a brain tumour.[93] A boy was operated for brain tumour. After the post checkups where the boy would be given Betapred. Four days after he had headaches and he vomited. He was sent to the hospital and was diagnosed with vomiting and did not suspect that it had to do with the treatment. The following day a doctor booked an ambulance for the boy to be operated for pressure relief. The boy became blind, and an MRI showed that damage had been done to the brain as a result of lack of oxygen. This damage was permanent.[94] When a man came into a hospital he was acting out sexually towards staff. He was later laid in the same room as a woman with anorexia and muscle weakness. The man raped her around 23:00 and the man was escorted out of the hospital in the morning.[95] A woman had esophageal cancer and the doctors offered to make her a new esophagus;

they did it with her stomach. In a checkup, a doctor discovered what he thought was rests of a cold in one of her lungs. She was booked the same examination and she did it twice more. She later was part of a research study in which she got an advanced PET X-ray in which suspspected tumours in her lung, inbetween the lungs, in the bronchi and in the pancreas was discovered. Two rounds of chemotherapy was done to her; her lips burst, she received blisters in the throat and she had to have a diaper. She was worried that the cancer had spread; as a part of a private health insurance she discovered that she had 13 metastasises in her brain. Later more metastases were discovered; she had them in her skeleton, eyes, and multiple internal organs organs. According to her doctors, nothing could be done, nothing could be done, however German doctors said that immununotherapy woul work for her condition. Imunotherapy requires medicine that is not approved of by Sweden; she had to do it privately. Her doctors changed their mind and they did six immunotherapy treatments; after the treatment she had no side effects and no cancer cells in her body.[96] A two-year old did not receive personal assistance for after having an operation after which she needed to breath through tubes. Their mootivation is that breathing is not a basic need according to *Försäkringskassan*.[97] A maternity clinic in Sollefteå closed and women must birth their children 20 miles away. A woman birthed her child in a car. There is six counties where women have to travel more than 30 miles to get to a hospital.[98] In 2014 a man discovered that he had prostate cancer. He was operated and survived, however four years later in 2018 he experienced pain in his whole body. It was ascertained that he had cancer in his whole torso. He only had six months left to live according to his doctor. Him and his wife planned to get him healthcare in Docrates, a private Finnish hospital; the doctor told them that they could get the same care in Sweden and dismissed the idea. At this time he had been through about seven Lutetium PSMA 177 treatments. After a scan, he still had cancer cells in his body.[99] The treatments removed the tumours, however it gave him side effects[100] such as damages to his bone marrow,[99] and him not being able to taste food; he lost tens of kilos.[100] A woman got stomach pains so she went to the healthcare center. She was then remited to the emergency room. In the waiting room she lost her seat when she went to the toilet and then she fainted. She was laid in the stomach departement.

It was already filled so she had her hospital bed in the corridor. She did not like how people went around her so she locked herself in a toilet; when she came back someone had taken her bed. She laid herself on a bunk and walked when she had energy. They started the examinations at five in the morning the next day, she had come at four the previous day.[101] A four year old had fever, vomiting and aches. He was sent home several times with pain relievers. In one visit, he ahd a wound on his hand and under his nose. At last he was diagnosed with leukemia.[102] A woman had cancer in the uterus and received an offer to get chemotherapy, but she wanted targeted radiation therapy. She went on her own accord and paid for the treatment in Finland. She wanted to get targeted radiation therapy before she went through chemotherapy. She became free from the cancer.[103]

2.3 Sweden during WW2

Sweden´s actions during World War II indicates they were on the German side. The Swedes negotiated with both sides and gave both of them resources, however by Germany the more resources with discounts aswell and other advantages. The Swedish attitude towards Jews during World War II and since World War II given how the Jews are treated in Sweden and Swedn´s politics regarding the Israel-Palestine conflict shows that they are not on side with the Jews.

Jews were treated badly from an individual perspective due to the arisation in areas like entrepeneurship and employment among others. There were two different types of citizenships: The A and the B citizenships. The Jews had the B citizneships and therefore their rights were not respected.[5 s.353] The Swiss and Swedes demanded the Germans to stamp red "J" in the passports of Jews. They did this for it to look like a German idea, however it came from Switzerland and Sweden.[5 s.294] Swedes risked their contacts in Germany if they amployed a Jew,[5 s.352] and therefore as an example the hospital director of Sweden did not allow young Jewish doctors to be employed in the hospitals of Stockholm during the end of the 1930s and during wartime,[5 s.349] and a Jewish woman was told that she could not be employed due to her being a Jew, and her man who was a barber was told the same.[5 s.352]

Due to the arisation there could be boycott of companies as well as loss of fiduciary duties, employment, informal ban of proffesion and discrimination in the labour market.[5 s.350] Germany demanded Sweden to be Aryanized due to the affairs between Germany and Sweden becoming more and more significant.[5 s.354] Swedish companies had to sign a contract that promised that the products were not to be sent further to Jewish companies.[5 s.359] The government did not react to these kinds of contracts.[5 s.360] German authorities demanded black lists from Swedish authorities, companies, people and information agencies to determine who companies and authoritties can do affairs with.[5 s.353] Swedsih companies started the Aryanization process on their own by cancelling their contacts with Swedish-Jewish companies and companies that had contact with Jewish interests, others reported Swedish non-Aryan companies and Geman commercial contacts if these still had contact with Jewish companies in Sweden trough decoys.[5 s.359]

A contemporary example to how Swedish Jews are suffering due to antisemitism is when an asylum seeking Palestininan was attacking a synagogue in Sweden with some other young men by throwing incendiaries; he was at first sentenced to prison and deportation. After an appeal, the court of appeal thought he would be treated badly in Israel and therefore repealed the decision, however they repeated the repeal because of impediment to enforcement.[5 s.319]

During the 1930s German Jews had money and valuables abroad. Sweden became a centre for selling those stolen valuables.[5 s.381] International Jewish organisations asked the Swedish Attorney General Herman Zetterberg for help to track Jewish belongings in Sweden in 1949. The government did not do anything. There were on four different occasions that Jewish organsiations asked for the same thing. In 1959 the Jewish assembly asked to postpone the prescription period for the Jewish belongings and also asked for the list over Jewish belongings; they did not receive what they asked for.[5 s.383] At last an investigation was set to search for Jewish belongings in Sweden. It started the 13 of February 1997 and ended after being postponed a few times in March of 1999.[5 s.381-382]

Olof Palme traveled to Algiers to meet the president of Algeria Boumedien,[5 s.29] however he was at a dinner with Yassir Arafat.[5 s.28] The meeting between the two were the day before Arafat was booked to hold a speech at UN about the interest of Palestine. Sweden was the only country that had voted for him to speak. Normally only representatives of member states and recognized states were allowed to speak at UN.[5 s.29] This was at a time when the Fatah-movement of Arafat still had genocide of Jews on their statutes.[5 s.30] The general consensus from the media newspapers were that Palme did not know that Arafat was at the meeting in advance[5 s.31] and *Expressen* went as far as to say that he had been tricked.[5 s.27]

When Palme lost the election in 1976, he became the vice chairman of *Socialistinternationalen*.[5 s.112] *Socialistinternationalen* had its intentions in supporting social democratic countries that tried to become better and become democratic. After an increase in socialist movements, the organisation lowered its demands and increased the amount of member states for example, they did not need to be democracies.[5 s.115]

The chancellor of Austria Bruno Kreisky, a political migrant in Sweden, had multiple minsiters that were Nazi during war time and one that participated actively in the killing of tens of thousands of Jews.[5 s.100] Kreisky met Arafat before Palme did.[5 s.99] Kreisky had suggested at a meeting for *Socialistinternationalen* to investiagte the conflict between Plaestine and Israel; Kreisky went to the midlle east at three occasions with Willy Brandt and Palme.[5 s.117] He said that it led to PLO and Arafat too be open for conversation.[5 s.117-118] Kreisky said that Israel could only exist as a crusader state.[5 s.116] In 1922 the Englishmen gave Israel to the UN and Emil Sandström was in charge. He proclaimed Israel as a state; five arab countries attacked Israel, all of them were UN countries.[5 s.206]

Bernadotte was a royalty, but were not next on the throne. He instead took on diplomatic mission such as that of mediate between the Israelites and the Paliestininans. He gave Jerusalem to the Arabs, made the Israeli airport Lydda and Israeli dock Haifa to a free dock and free airport and allowed free Jewish migration to Jerusalem for the coming two years after which the UN would take over.[5 s.202 & s.206] He were shot inn a car by Jewish terrorists when he were on his way to a meeting with the military of Jerusalem.[5 s.202] It was due to the sharing plan between Israel an Palestine that Folke Benadotte were killed by Israelites.[5 s.215]

Margot Wallström recognized Palestine as a state in 2014.[5 s.126] Sweden has been the biggest donator to the Palestinian state and was in 2018 the biggest donator per capita to UNWRA, the UN refugee agency for Palestinians.[5 s.28] The resolution 2334 by the UN in 2016 allowed countries, schools, universities and sport association to boycott Israel. Wallström accepted it and said it was important to set a foundation for further work in the security council. It would be a step towards the two-state-resolution according to her.[5 s.365]

The fleet Freedom Flotilla had eleven Swedes as well as the ship Mavi Marmara. Mavi Marmara had Turkish muslims that were part of the muslim brotherhood as well as IHH. Israeli soldiers borded the ship and killed nine men. They were condemned by Sweden, the EU as well as the rest of the world. There is evidence for Turkey to be involved in the incident. The fleet headed towards Gaza which was controlled by Hamas which belongs to the muslim brotherhood since the Israelites drew back from that region in 2005. Turkey who sailed Mavi Marmara is a member in Union of Good led by Shejk Youssef Qaradawi who has exclaimed that he wants to shoot the enemies of Allah, the Jews.[5 s.371-372]

Sweden let 250 000 German soldiers travel through Sweden in both directions.[5 s.339] When Finnland went to war with the Soviet Union, Sweden let German soldiers travel by Swedish railways to Finland.[5 s.339-340] German military supply ships sailed on Swedish water and German courier planes flew in Swedish airspaces. Sweden lit the lighthouses along the westcoasts as well as set up fairways. Swedish and German military set up mines in Östersjön to prevent the British fleet. Swedsih trucks laid up big amounts of ammunition and provisions.[5 s.340] The two long-term reasons for why Hitler wanted to invade Norway is to secure the border to the Atlantic ocean and to have submarine bases in Narvik nd to use these during submarine battles against England, however the short-term motive was to secure the transportation of Swdsih iron ore.[5 s.342]

There were about 1000 transactions between Swedn and Germany per day.[5 s.395] The receipts for Sweden´s foreign trades with Germany were put in archives and the amount of trade could be counted by shelf meters. Totally the receipts corresponded to 1 800 shelf meters.[5 s.396-397] While Sweden had affairs with both of the two warring parties, Sweden prioritised Germany by for instance giving them special sorts and discounts.[5 s.402] The total discount that Germany received was 29 percent.[5 s.410] Swedes were allowed to work in Germany and German were allowed to work in Sweden.[5 s.404]

Sweden´s exports of machines, metalls, minerals, paper and wood to Germany increases during wartime. The exportation of ball bearings are the most essential for Germany and it borke the rules of the Swedish and British agreement to keep it at the same rate or at a lower rate as before the war throughout the war.[5 s.407] The Swedish ball bearings industry dominated 70 percent of the world market.[5 s.408]

The United States wanted Sweden to reduce the amount of ball bearings Sweden exported to Germany to a third of the 1943 levels; Sweden refused. Sweden was dependant on the US for oil, Germany could only give Sweden seven percent of its consumption.[5 s.412] Sweden invalidated the ball bearings contract with Germany due to transportation problems, but Sweden had subsidiaries in Germany that could provide for Germany´s ball bearing´s need. Sweden increased the amount of ball bearing stell to 20 820 tonnes in 1944 from 12 600 tonnes that Sweden had exported between 1941-1943. Sweden also increased the amount of machines they exported by 200 percent in 1944 in comparison to 1943.[5 s.413]

The Swedish iron ore were 18 percent of the iron ore that Germany received and it was of a higher quality than other types.[5 s.429] Between 1939 and 1940 Sweden gave 40 percent of Germany´s iron ore, but for 1941 it decreased to 25 percent.[5 s.430] In 1942 the US released 30 000 tonnes of oil in excahange for Sweden to release two norweigan ships with ball bearings to England; Sweden released its ships a year later.[5 s.431] In an agreement Sweden would stop escorting German ships on Östersjön, reduce the ball bearing export, iron ore export and stop letting German troops transport themselves on Swedish land in exchange from Sweden receiving more oil and rubber; Sweden accepted it while not living up to their part of the agreement.[5 s.432] Even if Swedish exportation of Ball bearings reduced, the Germans ball bearing factories in Schweinfurt who was a subsidiary to SKF owned by *Skandinaviska Enskila Banken* owned by the family Wallenberg.[5 s.433]

2.4 It is all about *Folkhemmet*

The greatest threat to the Swedes is the fact that the politicians wants to control the healthcare with giving staff big amounts of paper work aswell as guidelines for treatments instead of letting doctors treat the patient according to his needs. It denies the elderly the care that they need and therefore resulting in deaths.

During the World War II era Sweden gave ideas as well as supported the Germans, however their fake neutrality has left the Swedes with something not to feel shame about. During the first part of the Covid-19 pandemic, Anders Tegnell was well proud of the results of the herd immunity strategy, but only a few months in started denying that Sweden had such a strategy; he managed to mitigate the incoming criticisms for Sweden´s strategy as well as its legacy there on after.

While Adolf Hitler had inspirations from Rudolf Kjellén and his geopolitical stance; Kjellén saw the international arena as a fight between states from a darwinistic point of view likewise did the

nazis.[5 s.223] Kjelléns imperialistic views may have been nationalistic while the nazis´ views were racial. They were nontheless similar because of Karl Haushofer who was interested in Kjellén introduced Hitler to Kjelléns ideas when Hitler was in prison.[104]

3.1 How Sweden corona handled in the beginning

On the 16th of January Tegnell said that the world has capacity to handle the virus in a good way to prevent its progress and he said that it was likely that some people would be infected with the virus when answering the question whether corona would come to Europe.[Sveriges radio 2020 referneced in 105] On the 20th January he said that it would be unlikely for Sweden to have a spread.[Dawod 2020 referenced 105] In mid-February the WHO said that it is uncertain whether the pandemic will even out[106]. Tegnell wanted to delay the corona strategy until cases in Sweden started to pop up,[107] even though Tegnell welcomed people from Italy and other corona-stricken countries early 2020.

Tegnell claimed that the corona virus does not have an effective ability for transmission between humans on January the 16th.[Sveriges radio refernced in 105] He repeated it on the 20th and said that it would need to spread to the healthcare for it to be deemed as effective.[Dawod refernced in 105] It is more likely to be infected indoors than outdoors and door handle is not something to worry about because viruses does not thrive in sunlight according to

Tegnell.[TT 2020 refernced in 105] He says that you have to be close to someone for a long time[Nordevik & TT 2020 A refernced in 105] When SAS stopped all flights to north Italy on the 3rd March, Tegnell did not agree with the decision and said that it is not well-grounded in medical facts. He said that Corona is not asymptomatic on the 3rd of March,[Brischetto 2020 refernced in 105] even though Lena Einhorn warned him after reading that people without obvious symptoms can spread the infection,[108] but on the 5th of April, he changed his mind and said that small non-significant group, ten percent of infected, are asymptomtic and that they do not matter for the spread of infection.[Nordevik & TT 2020 S refernced in 105]

When students came home from the holiday that is located around week nine in 2020 a few more countries than China had corona virus outbreaks. *Folkhälsomyndigheten* did not see any reasons from an infection control perspective for students without symptoms having distance education because Tegnell said that there is nothing that says that corona is asymptomatic. The director of education Lena Holmdahl said that if students are at home because of worry, it will be considered invalid absence. It was a single school that had a different policy, and it was that students that had been in China quarantined for 14 days.[109] Eleven planes from Italy landed in late February from the holidays, but according to the infection control physician Per Follin it is not a worry since the ski resorts and the airports is not risk factors, however Follin and Tegnell encourages people to contact 1177 if they show symptoms.[110] It was the holidays in February 2020 that was responsible for the general societal spread and lead to the spread in the elderly home according to *Coronakommisionen*.[111] A person that stayed in Wuhan for five hours was told to quarantine for 14 days by China. When he contacted *Smittskydd Skåne*, they said that as long as he did not have any symptoms, he could come home and if he received symptoms within 14 days, he should contact a doctor.[112] There is no reason for closing the borders according to Tegnell because ""Closing borders, in my opinion, is ridiculous, because COVID-19 is in every European country now""[113] and ""I think open border are always a good idea""[114, translated qoute]. On January the 16th Tegnell said that people could travel to China, and that they should be careful hand hygiene.[Sveriges Radio 2020 refernced 105] The persons that comes home to Sweden was recommended to have a quarantine, but not they were not obligated to.[Gilda 2020 referenced in 105]

When SAS stooped its direct flights to Beijing and Shanghai, Air China continued and increased the flights by five departures. Tegnell claimed that health checkups not to be necessary with flights from China to Sweden because there is no direct flights between China and Sweden which is not true. His claims came from an interview and claimed that the qoutes from him were innacurate, and that they were only talking about Wuhan and not China in general, meaning he claimed that there were no direct flights to Wuhan. He stills claims that SAS is the only flight company that does direct flights to China though and it is not true because Air China does it as well. Tegnell also claimed that the whole thing is meaningless because most of the tourists from China dooes not come via direct flights[115]. Tegnell does not want health checkups on airport because it is inneffective, he instead wants passengers to listen to information and contact the healthcare in case of symptoms.[116] Untill late March there are still no health checkups on airports. It is authorities who decides if there is going to be checkups or not.[117] *Folkhälsomyndigheten* does not want to enforce health checkups due to the process of the checkup being time consuming and they think that only a few of them will carry the virus.[118] The airline *SAS* decided to stop flights to north Italy early March 2020; Tegnell commented on it and said that the decision is not based on facts.[119] Tegnell did not think all of the corona cases came from the Alps, but from the US hence probably why he did not think of health checkups on airports.[120] *Folkhälsomyndigheten* did not think it was necessary to make people who came back from Iran and Italy to go into quarantine. They would rather have them live normal life because they can trace infection easier.[121]

Tegnell thought that Corona would be as lethal as influenza and last as long as an influenza period which is eight to ten weeks, he said this th first of February[122] while Anthony Fauci a month later claimed Covid-19 would become ten times more lethal than influenza.[123] Mia Bryting, a microbiologist at *Folkhälsomyndigheten* said that we would reach the peak in February or March 2020[122] while Fauci said that Covid-19 only had started.[123]

As soon as on the 15th of March 2020 Tegnell claimed that Sweden has reached its peak and that the amount of cases might rise slightly, but it will eventually go down.[124] In the beginning of March 2020, Tegnell said that if we could wait until the summer, then we could get rid of corona altogether.[125]

Tegnell did not think that corona would spread further outside of China and therefore,[121] but when the reusult came, Tegnell realised that too many elderly people had died. The group that *Folkhälsomyndigheten* wanted to protect.[126]

Tegnell said that the success of dealing with the winter influenza in 2020 made the corona death toll high the same year.[127]

3.2 How Sweden recieved a natural herd immunity strategy

There were three strategies that were as options in the early planning: a quarantine for four weeks in the beginning, huge amounts of infection tracing and placing the infected in a two week quarantine or the natural herd immunity strategy. When the mails about the herd immunity strategy leaked Tegnell said that it was not about sacrificing humans and that the herd immunity strategy was the only feasible option.[128] He says that the only way of stopping a pandemic is to reach an immunity in the population[129] and he has also said that the immunity would come before the vaccine,[130 30:23-30:34] despite the claims about a natural herd immunity being superior to other strategies he has also said that herd immunity through a spread of infection has not the been the main strategy, he said that the strategy is to have a slow enough spread for the healthcare to have a reasonable peace of mind. He adds that the two are goals are not contradictory and that herd immunity is good as a concept.[131]

The inspiration for the natural herd immunity strategy came from the former state epidemiologist Johan Giesecke. Giesecke was the state epidemiologist from 1995 to 2005 and he was the pesrson that recruited Tegnell. Giesecke emailed with personalities of *Folkhälsomyndigheten* and in the first mail he told them that the virus is more contagious than influenza and would infect everybody in two months. He said that most would not notice that they were infected and the ones who would get sick would only receive a cold. He said that the of the elderly so that the health care would not suffer. He predicted that the time where there would be most sick in hospitals would be within three to four weeks. He said that people under the age of 60 would work from home as a start and then go back when the situation is over.[132]

Giesecke proposed that *Folkhälsomyndigheten* would make a graph for corona showcasing the deaths in an email and compare it to influenza and instructed them to use the graph used for the influenza for 2018-2019 and Anders Wallensten thought it would be a good idea. Someone in *Folkhälsomyndigheten* wrote that it would not be smart to come out with ""quick and dirty resultat"" because people would not be less concerned if they showed that corona is less mortal than influenza and suggested they would have several factors in their graph.[132]

Tegnell offered Giesecke a work opportunity, Giesecke accepted it. The first proposal Gesecke gave was to drop the measure of closing college schools and university saying it does not have an epidemiological effect and that it would bring hope to the public. He mailed the leading infection control physician Preben Aavitsland Norway´s strategy is wrong. Giesecke officially signed a contract and worked as a consultant and would receive at a maximum of 800 hours with 1250 Swedish crowns an hour. Even though Giesecke has appear in media, the media does not know that he works for *Folkhälsomyndigheten.* His purpose is to help the unit with analysis and support them in their work with modeling and analysis of covid-19. Tegnell is the person who Giesecke mails to the most and Tegnell is the most efficient with mailing Giesecke out of everyone he mails. Tegnell mails Jan Albert the most. Giesecke signs a *jäv*-declaration. He misspelt his name, does not fill in his previous job and does not fill in an assignment of relative which should be filled in. With his new job he gives his wife contacts with financiers. Tegnell and Giesecke kept contact during the summer 2020.[132]

On the 19th of March Tegnell mails Giesecke if the spread of the virus reduces when the immunity increases or if the spread stops when herd immunity is achieved. The former state epidemiologist Annika Linde writes a Facebook post where she says that it would be beneficial if students of young ages and their parents would have a slow spread of the virus and that it is the strategy that *Folkhälsomyndigheten* is going with.[133]

Tegnell said to *Dagens Nyheter* that natural herd immunity is not the ambition, but rather the ambition is to have a slow enough spread so that the health care. Tegnell read a mail from an old person who suggested that Sweden would handle corona within the younger generation the way they did with Varicella. The person suggested that the hotels would be booked for the younger people since they will be empty anyway and the spread of infection would make it so that they do not have to vaccinate themselves meaning they would create herd immunity. The people in the hotel would volunteer under controlled forms and not meet with sensitive humans. There would also be a huge group that would work and study for free. Tegnell got inspired and suggested it would be a good idea to hold the schools open. He discussed the matter with Mika Salminen which said that he had thought about the idea already. Salminen said that the attack rate on the elderly will be reduced by 10% if the proposal is put in place and Tegnell said that it seems worth it, however early august 2020 Tegnell said that holding the schools open was about a possible rather than expected effect and it was not because of immunity.[133]

Linde wrote an email to Tegnell regarding herd immunity and said that she realised that Sweden did not gain immunity. Linde said that corona could not avoid immunity like influenza can do and she mentioned that the fact that children mostly are asymptomatic it can help with the immunity. Tegnell has constantly said that the asymptomatic feature is not a thing with corona. She also said that the immunity gained with this method would make the pressure on the healthcare lessen and it would help until they would have more health care resources and hopefully a vaccine. Tegnell thanked her for the thoughts but did not agree with her thinking that children would play a role of being an engine in the pandemic, though he said that they had done a good job during the week of the vacations to Italy[133] where Tegnell wanted Sweden to catch corona cases in Sweden. On the 24th of February during week 9 in 2020 which is a holiday for students Tegnell criticised that Italy has invested in cancelling flights and have control over their borders. He said that Sweden´s strategy of trying to catch the virus inside the country was a far better strategy.[130] 07:52-08:00

Tegnell commented on how Great Britain handled the corona strategy which was through herd immunity in mid-March. The immunity was thought to come when 40 million Brits had been infected. Tegnell said that Sweden is doing something similar and that it follows a more scientific strategy. The strategy is about having a flat curve meaning having the corona cases be similar from day to day instead of having peaks.[134] During the time when Tegnell denied that Sweden has had a herd immunity strategy Tegnell has constantly said that the spread of infection must lay under a line which represent the capacity for the healthcare.[135] The Swedish ambassador for America Karin Ulrika Olofsdotter said that Sweden wanted to keep the spread of infection below the line in which the Swedish healthcare system would not collapse.[136] 01:22-01:28 The told strategy has not been the same, but the actual strategy has been the same throughout. Tegnell had deleted over 200 mails from January to April.[137] *Folkhälsomyndigheten* said in response to that that it was by an individual employee[138] and Tegnell said they were not relevant for recording[139] and that they were probably discussions with different groups[140] or working material, and the deletion of mails were important for economic reasons. The Media lawyer Jeanette Gustafsdotter says that if it is mails who has affected the decisions that the authority has taken it is misconduct. The missing mails were between Tegnell, experts and authority employees. *Folkhälsomyndigheten* says that it is Tegnell that has deleted the mails, but he has no memory of it. Eight out of all the mails that *Folkhälsomyndigheten* has given out were coated with secrecy because they were mails with the foreign.[140]

The authority *Folkhälsomyndigheten* thought that a natural herd immunity via enough people catching the virus and becoming sick would defeat the virus,[130 29:28-29:57] however the prime minister said on the 15th of January 2021 that Sweden has not had a strategy that involves herd immunity[130 38:18-38:28] and in March 2020 Lena Hallengren denied that Sweden had a herd immunity strategy.[120]

Sweden has not had a lockdown. Some reasons are that Tegnell thought that Sweden peaked in corona cases[141] and therefore a lockdown strategy probably was never planned for, Tegnell predicted that the hered immunity would come before the vaccine[130 30:23-30:34] and since a herd immunity strategy requires a slight spread in the population, a lockdown would shut it down. He has said that with a lockdown, the corona cases increases greatly during non-lockdown periods and it would not be a benifit to a herd immunity strategy.

Tegnell had a prediction that China was going handle the virus and it did not end up like that and therefore Tegnell and *Folkhälsomyndigheten* probably did not plan for the pandemic adequately.[142] When corona cases kept increasing, he came to the conlusion that corona would not be a classic pandemic, he rather concluded that ther would be a few hot spots. The infection toll was 180.[143] Another reason is that Tegnell thought that an immunity among the population would reduce the amount of cases during Autumn 2020.[144]

The authority *Folkhälsomyndigheten* thought that a natural herd immunity would develop in the population.[130 29:29-29:57] Because of the natural herd immunity, Tegnell did not want the vaccine early in the pandemic and on the 17th of March 2020 he said that a lot speaks for the vaccine being too far away because you need a vaccine that works and therefore will the herd immunity come first in the population[130 10:23-30:34] and in April he claimed that Sweden would gain a higher immunity before receiving the vaccine, however four months later in August he said that an immunity only reduces the spread and not that it completely stops the spread.[133]

Tegnell started to assert that the Swedish people had an immunity and that it people would be outside more in the summer; he said that the weather during the summer and the amount of immune people would lower the spread of infection suggesting that he was not worried about people going outside and spreading the virus.[130] [30:36-30:44] *Folkhälsomyndigheten* had the mathematician Tom Britton that counted on herd immunity. He showed in a graph that if 90% of the population would become infected then 20% of the population would become immune.[130] [30:44-30:49] Britton also mentioned the 20th of April 2020 that in a month meaning in May 2020 that most of the spread of the disease in Stockholm had already been and Stockhholm would reach that herd immunity.[130] [30:52-31:01]

On the 9th of May when we could test immunity Tegnell said this:

> "We are now getting results from several countries showing that our Nordic neighbours maybe one to two percent of the population are now immune while the estimate from Sweden is around twenty-five percent. So of course, we are much further into the epidemic and much closer to having a level of immunity in the population and that we have very clearly keep a low number of cases everyday while having a very open society. "[130] [31:11-31:40] translated qoute

In the middle of April 2020, Tegnell was sure that the level of immunity would affect the spread of infection.[130 31:01-31:05] as an example Tegnell claimed that you are immune to Corona for six months if you recceived the diagnosis and said that you can be with people during that time even people in risk groups.[145] Before starting to test immunity, Tom Britton and Anders Tegnell predicted the immunity in the country would be 20. 30 or 40 percent, however after the tests on the 20th of May 2020, it came out that the Stockholm region had 7,3 percent, the region Västra Götaland had 3,7 percent and the region Skåne had 4,2 percent. The reaction to the results from Britton was that he said that him and others would go back to the desk.[130 31:51-32:15]

In May 2020 Tom Britton said that Stockholm could reach herd immunity in a month meaning June. Earlier forecasts stated that 60 percent of the population needed to be infected for the population to reach herd immunity. Britton stated that only 40 to 45 percent of the population needed to be infected if the reproduction number is 2,5 meaning that every new case infects 2,5 persons on average. It is Britton and Pieter Trapman that are behind the new forecast. Britton said that the positive thing with this model is that Sweden only needed few restrictions. Anders Tegnell verifies Brittons prognosis about Stockholm reaching immunity in June.[146] Tom Britton said in April 2020 that half of the population in Stockholm would be infected by the end of May 2020. He said in December the same year that he was wrong because he assumed that corona would behave like influenza, did not think about behaviour and restrictions and did not include cluster infection. He still claimed that herd immunity was possible. He claimed that him saying that herd immunity was possible did not affect the behaviour of people. He hopes that Sweden would gain immunity via vaccination.[147] conjunction with him correcting his previous statements, he said that 15 percent of the population in Sweden is immune and that mass vaccinations would establish herd immunity. He thought that half of Sweden would have antibodies by the second half of the spring 2021 because of vaccines and because of being infected and receiving antibodies. Another miscalculation from him was that he thought that the gained herd immunity in the population would decrease a second wave. He said that it was partially true.[148] Tom Britton received the prize for the statistics promoter of the year for the year 2020.[149]

3.3 Why Herd immunity would not be a viable strategy

A woman had mild symptoms of Covid-19 and tested positive for it on the 17th of April. On the 2nd May she tested negative, however she received symptoms once again and got her positive test result on the 3rd of July suggesting that immunity towards Covid-19 falls off quickly and that herd immunity would not be viable strategy.[150] A healthcare worker who has had the two planned doses of covid-19 vaccines and one booster first had a Covid-19 infection with the delta variant to then 20 days later have an infection with the Omicron variant. The Omicron variant can evade immunity from past infections further suggesting a natural herd immunity strategy is useless.[151] When Tegnell speculated about how herd immunity would play out in Sweden, he suggested that if 60% of the population would become infected, only about four to six percent would need hospital care; as of the last day that Covid-19 was recognised a pandemic the 31st of March 2022 18 412 people died of corona out of 2 487 967 Covid cases in total which means 7,40042 ‰ of infected people died of the disease.[152]

3.4 The actual strategy

Sweden has since the 1990s had a significant migration and dealt with many issues because of it. The beginnning of the pandemic were not an exception as the architect himself Tegnell were not against movements between countries. This with the combination of late and weak measures increased the Covid cases early.

Tegnell and *Folkhälsomyndigheten* was proud at first of the herd immunity strategy and made ridiculous statements regarding its consequences. He later told everyone Sweden did not have a herd immunity strategy, however the strategy itself did not switch up. The most signifiacnt measure put by *Folkhälsomyndigheten* was to recommend face masks in the public transport.

The thing I found the most bizarre is that Tegnell´s description of the intent with the Swedish startegy. In the beginning he said that we had to have a flat curve meaning the spread of infection being consistent. When he later change the descriptiojn of the Swedish strategy he explained that the goal is for the spread of infection to be consistently below the full capacity of the healthcare meaning the healthcare would be able to take care of all patients.

4.1 The Sweden image

The sterilization program was not a secret to the public. It was rather that Sweden wanted to be the envy of the world.[3] Presently Sweden wants to stand out in world.

During Autumn 2020 Tegnell claimed that Swedes kept following recommendations while *Telia, MSB* and *Novus* made reports that it was not the case. According to critics Tegnell did not warn the public enough for the season of Autumn and when he commented on it, he did not say that he or them was wrong, rather he said that it was about the signals that it sends because he did not want to worry the public too much.[153] This is due to the way that the Swedish politicians wants to portray Sweden, they want *Sverigebilden*, the Swedish picture, to be positive. The effort to spread positivity about Sweden to the world came from debates in other countries about migration and criminality.[154] Sweden arranged a new authority whose purpose was to defend Sweden from outside "non-truths" according to the Swedish government.[155] It was the site *Sweden.se* run by Swedish institutions such as the Government Offices that posted pictures of smiling politicians that talks about how good it is in Sweden. The attorney general Morgan Johansson said that if Sweden can manage the jobs, school and housing while reducing social gaps then they can manage and prevent criminality. He claims that Sweden can manage jobs[154] while Sweden has the sixth highest unemployment rate.[156] In Sweden there is so called *no-go zones* where ambulance staff are afraid of going because it is dangerous places. The twitter account of the ministry of foreign affairs said that Sweden has 53 places where there is crime, social worries and insecurity which are falsely called *no-go*-zones.[155] The methods for saving the Swedish picture is not only online. Swedish ambassadors are pressed to talk about Sweden and say that the Swedish corona strategy is the same as other countries with some exceptions.[157] The minister of foreign affairs claimed that the only way that Sweden is different in comparison to other countries is that Sweden does not close schools and preschool and does not implement lockdowns and she also claims that Sweden did not have a herd immunity strategy. Lena Hallengren claimed that the Swedish health care has survived and that there has always been between 20 to 30 percent available hospital beds and that people that has needed advanced care has received it[158]. Johan Carlsson said that Själland had a lot of corona cases and Skåne had few, however the death toll per citizen was the same in the areas and Skåne had more patients and more who used intensive care than Denmark, he then claimed that it was not because of the Swedish measures.[159] Tegnell has said that personal relations does not affect the decisions of *Folkhälsomyndigheten*, however he did not mention that Johan Carlsson received a mail from Giesecke where Giesecke suggested that they should drop the measure about distance education in universities and colleges and gymnasiums.[132] When countries started to ease restrictions, Tegnell said that they were following the Swedish model and said that it made them confident and motivated.[160] On April 21st *Folkhälsomyndigheten* put out a report that stated that a third of Stockholm´s residents would be infected by corona by 1st May. They withdrew it. The report had as a starting point that every corona case would infect 999 other persons.[161] Ann Linde(So) insisted that Sweden did not use a herd immunity strategy in April 2020[162] and her response early June 2020 to the foreign medias claiming Sweden does use herd immunity was that Sweden she wanted to be clear that Sweden does not use herd immunity.[158] Lena Hallengren(So) said that the only two ways that

Sweden has acted differently is by not closing schools and not demanding people to stay at home.[163] The Swedish ambassador to the UK Torbjörn Sohlström claimed that Sweden did not use herd immunity.[164] Misse Wester, a proffesor of risk management and public safety thinks that Swedish authorities have performed well because of they have been through many crises and ignores the obvious faults authorities have done, especially *Folkhälsomyndigheten.* She also thinks that the small differences in statements between *Folkhälsomyndigheten* and independant infection control doctor is not significant enogh while they actually do because the differences can result in diverse outcomes.[165] While Sweden was the 10th worst country considering deaths per capita from Covid-19 Thomas Erdbrink and Christina Anderson wrote about how amazing Sweden´s strategy was and rewarding Sweden for being unique.[166] About a year after Covid-19 started Tegnell did not think Sweden could do better tostop the spread of infection.[167]

4.2 Censoration

It was already the 27th of January 2020 that Christer Jansson at *Folkhälsomyndigheten* contacted *MSB*. Their contact is used to report citizens to the security service who are critical towards the pandemic strategy. It is a person from *Folkhälsomyndigheten* who writes an email to a person at *MSB* about people on the internet who devalues the Swedish pandemic strategy. A person who was frustrated about Sweden not closing borders and comparing it to other countries that did was registered as an agent of foreign power by *Folkhälsomyndigheten*. They register "false rumors" from posts and considers blocking the user or delete posts. Christer Jansson says that he does not remember the mails between him and the person at *MSB*.[168] This is similar to how doctor Li Wenliang was treated by the Chinese government. The doctor discovered the new coronavirus in one of his patients which had gluacoma. He decided to post about the case and advice fellow doctors to wear protective clothing. He then had to sign a letter where he stated that he had spread false rumours. If he would not; he would have been arrested and tried in a court of law.[169] Doctors who have insisted people to wear facial masks have been reprimanded or fired. Brusselaers was publicly reprimanded by her department chair and was called ""troublemaker"" and ""a danger to society"". Her colleague said that they had to defend and be loyal to *Folkhälsomyndigheten*. an ophthalmologist Agnieszka Howoruszko wore a face mask while working with patients at the regional hospital in Landskrona and was reprimanded twice by her manager. Howoruszko protested and the eye clinic was the only one to allow the clinic's doctors to wear facial masks, however other staff could not wear facial masks, in the entire province.[108] The union *Komunnal* reported *Arbetsmiljöverket* because *Arbetsmiljöverket* subdued their demands of facial masks. *Arbetsmiljöverket* subdued the demand because they did not want to deviate from the opinion of *Folkhälsomyndigheten* about facial masks. No unions or safety representatives was allowed to be in the process and they apologised to *Kommunal* for feeling ignored. The medical expert of *Arbetsmiljöverket* came to the conclusion that face shields alone is not enough, however it was silenced and was not included in the pronouncement of the court. Instead it was said that one should determine locally if face shield was enough.[170] When *svt* took part of an internal mail from *Arbetsmiljöverket* where it was revealed that they took part with *Folkhälsomyndigheten* to not be in a difficult situation where different authorities have different statements and to avoid difficult debates. The mails were later deleted.[171]

In a debate article, Victor Malm shames Lena Einhorn for criticizing Tegnell. He says that she can not say that the Swedish strategy is an experiment because every country's corona strategy is a strategy.[172] When a group demonstrated in central Stockholm, they were spat on by passers-by.[173] When the nurse Latifa Löfvenberg came out in media and told about the oxygen situation, she was fired and the reason for it was not given.[174] Uppsala municipality did not want to give out information about which retirement homes that were stricken by corona and motivated the silence by saying that they do not want to increase the worry within the public.[175] When *Folkhälsomyndigheten* received critique for their strategy in their mail, the titles to news medias were about giving *Folkhälsomyndigheten* police protection. When 50 000 mails were examined, only about 80 of them could be seen as hate and the rest were critique.[176] An investigation showed that Swedish news medias were slow to critique *Folkhälsomyndigheten* and the Swedish pandemic strategy while foreign medias were faster. It took Swedish medias until the summer 2020 to start to criticize the strategy.[177] The graph for the death toll that *Svt* had in their program *Rapport* changed the scale so that it looked like the

death toll did not change as much as it did.[178]
When the newspaper *Ekuriren* demanded the
regions and municipalities to about the death toll
and infection rate for corona, they were at first
willing to do it, however a month later they
refused due to secrecy. After an appeal from
Ekuriren, the municpalities Nyköping, Eskilstuna,
Oxelösund, Katrineholm, Gnesta och Vingåker
became transparent. The municiaplites Flen and
Strängnäs still did not want to be transparent about
their death toll and infection rate.[179] Irene
Svenonius(Mo) said that everyone that seeks
intensive care received it, however a conslutant at
the hospital Karolinska claimed that they have
denied a number of patients due to lack of staff,
premises and equipment.[180] Cecilia Söderberg
Naucler critiqued *Folkhälsomyndigheten* along
with other scientists in an article in *Svenska
Dagbladet*, mentioning that if Great Britain would
use Sweden´s Covid strategy, it could have led to
250 000 more deaths and another statistic using
simulations to know how lockdowns and the
closing of schools would affect the spread of
infection; Sweden was the only country to have an
R value over one meaning that every new infection
would hypothetically lead to at least one more
infection. Sweden was also the only country that

had not introduced school closing and lockdowns at the time. They critiqued the fact that only people with symptoms are recommended to stay at home despite asymptomatics.[181] In another article in *Aftonbladet* Söderberg Naucler stated she wanted to resign as he does not listen to the whole world of scientists. She mentions multiple misjudgements and the fact that *Folkhälsomyndigheten* denies powerful measures as unsecure and further she wants a lockdown in Sweden,[182] however despite her many criticisms of *Folkhälsomyndigheten* she decided to come out and say that she actually did not want Tegnell to resign[183] and *Folkhälsomyndigheten* mapped healthcare resources the in each of the regions. *Dagens Nyheter* wanted to take part in thenumbers regarding isolation capacity and the number of intensive care beds in isolation in each of the regions, however *Socialstyrelsen* told *Dagens nyheter* that the information was under secrecy and could therefore not give them the information they wanted.[184]

4.3 The elderly

The government´s real strategy for the elderly was revealed by a government document that discussed the economic consequences of a predicted Covid death toll. It stated that if 2 000 more pensioners dies in 2020 and the deaths are evenly distributed throughout the year then the government will save 152 000 000 sek. It also was stated that if 2021 starts with 2 000 less pensioners then the government will save 306 000 000 sek.[185 p.64-65] Similarly Giesecke stated that with a herd immunity startegy the frail and old population will die first and then the death toll will reduce.[186]

Corona came into the elderly care because the general spread of the infection was high[187 24:51-25:10] which came as a result of people coming home during the holidays week nine 2020[111] and it was potentially the staff with asymptomatic spread that spread the virus because the virus was still in the elderly care during the visitation ban.[187 24:51-25:10] The measures taken by the municipality was to introduce visitation ban in the elderly care the 1st of April 2020 which was introduced two weeks prior to what *Folkhälsomyndigheten* recommended,[187 14:48-14:53] and short-term places where the infected elderly can live and to implement Covid-team in the home care.[187 21:18-21:29] The Covid-teams goes home to the elder in need of care against Corona.[188]

There were a lot of demerits regarding the staff, there were a lot of different staff in the elderly care[187 11:45-11:47] resulting in a lot of new persons going in and out of the home which increases the chance of the spread of infection. There were too many temporary posts, low level of education, low level of the Swedish language and few assistant nurses.[187 23:23-23:34] The staff that had temporary posts had to be scheduled in a way that they had right to sickness benefit for them not to come to the job if they had symptoms.[187 24:23-24:36] Newly educated assistant nurses must work 731 days to be able to receive a permanent employment while non-educated person receives spots. A lot of retirement home staff in the municipality of Oskarshamn has low language skills that results in misunderstandings. There is no language test, but an assessment is done, and it is put in the context for the individual.[189]

The healthcare has had complications with the elderly, it mostly regards individual assessments which was made on 80% of the Covid-sick[187 03:05-03:10] and most of the individual assessments was made by phone.[187 03:10-03:18] When 847 Covid-patients in the elderly care was analysed only about 5 to 7 percent of them received a physical individual assessment.[187 30:44-31:03] In the region of Västra Götaland they have had the medically responsible nurse physically with the patient while the doctor is in a video call with them.[187 31:37-32:02] There is also a problem regarding medical records because they are double written.[187 31:28-31:33]

As of the 18th of May 2020, 90 percent of the people that had died were 70 or older and half of them was in special accommodation and died there[190] and 90 percent of elderly was not sent to the hospital and was left to die at the retirement homes.[191] The people that live in special accommodation have small medical margins. *Socialstyrelsen* has repeatedly said that the elderly should be treated in the retirement homes, however they are not for medical check-ups and a lot of the people die because they do not receive correct assessment and therefore does not receive basic care. The positives with medical care in hospitals is oxygen, nutrient drip, thrombosis prophylaxis and close monitoring which is usually not available outside the hospital, or there is no medically competent person who prescribes. Palliative care is prescribed without careful medical assessment and sometimes without the doctor seeing the elderly patient. Geriatrician Yngve Gustafson has criticized the medical profession because of their lack of knowledge when it comes to drug treatment of the elderly, it is serious because the number one for disease is improper use of drugs. About 70 percent of the elderly that were taken care of in hospitals survived. In the elderly homes the infection control competence and a lot of elderly dies because of a lack of nutrition. A lack of nutrition leads to a weak immune system.[190] In 2017 about 40 000 elderly suffered from lack of nutrition and about 100 000 risked to be suffering from lack of nutrition. Accrording to Yngve Gustaffson, the elderly needs people to sit down with them so that they eat enough of what they need and Åsa Regner says that dietists are needed to increase the awareness of the elders´ diets.[192] It is not a new phenomenon because it has been like this during periods with winter sickness. The elderly care generally has low medical skills, low staffing, and nursing homes are not suitable for barrier care.[190] An 81-year-old was denied respirator because their healing ability was not enough to do it.[193] Between 16 and 22 percent of elderly patients did not receive doctor assessments in person and 40 percent of the persons not receiving a doctor's assessment did not receive an assessment from a nurse either. The persons who received their assessments per distance received it through telephone.[194]

4.4 Systemic complications

Sweden has a system based upon four levels: The EU makes decision that affects the regions and the municipalities, the state are affected by the government that makes proposition meaning bills that the parliament must vote through, the regions that takes care of the healthcare system, the municipalities that has control over schools, elderly car and social services and there is also authorities that takes care of different thing such as *Folkhälsomyndigheten* that works as Sweden´s own *WHO* or *Försäkringskassan* who takes care of social insurances.[195] The problem is that there are politicians in the municipality of Stockholm that wants the municipality to employ doctors to the elderly care.[187 38:08-38:14] The authority *Folkhälsomyndigheten* has been the biggest decider when it comes to how the pandemic was to be handled because the prime minister gave them the responsibility, but they did not know about the flaws of the elderly care.[187 03:558-04:13]

In the municipality of Göteborg a lot of employees experienced that they were not allowed to work at home even though that they could and that it was a recommendation from *Folkhälsomyndigheten*. The director for the municipality thinks that workers are needed at their workplace and should be their as long as they are not sick.[196]

When corona restrictions started to ease in May 2021, Norbotten was the area with the most amount of spread of infection in Europe. The infection control physician Anders Nystedt wanted to keep the restrictions instead of easing them, however *Folkhälsomyndigheten* kept to the plan and eased the restrictions in Norrbotten with the rest of the country.[197]

4.5 Government crisis

A government crisis is when a political party in the government does not want to be in the government anymore. There has been three during the pandemic because of following matters: Migration, Oil refinery expansion, an expansion of Arlanda, a change in the rules of order and market rents.

The reason for *Miljöpartiet* wanting to leave the government was because *Socialdemokraterna* wanted to lower immigration numbers,[198] however they started to demand other things in combination with it; the demands were to stop Preem´s expansions due to the environment[199] and the expansion of Arlanda.[198]

Socialdemokraterna negotiated with the four political parties that was once in the political coalition called *Alliansen* about migration. Only two of the parties are in the government; *Liberalerna* and *Centerpartiet* while the other two; *Kristdemokraterna* and *Moderaterna* is in the opposition. It was *Miljöpartiet* did not approve of it, but the problem was that it was not possible for the leading political party, *Socialdemokraterna* to build a majority with the two left political parties. The migration policies that *Miljöpartiet* is against is: There should be a volume target for how many asylum seekers there should be, the prescription will be doubled from four to eight years and there a sharpening of maintenance requirements. The alternative that is being discussed within *Miljöpartiet* is to leave the government if the party does not accept the settlement, however it is not final.[198]

When the parliament were meant to bring forth a new asylum legislation that would be applied during Spring of 2021, *Miljöpartiet* threatened with leaving the government, if *Socialdemokraterna* would introduce their new restrictive legislation.[199] Stefan Löfven has constantly said that the migration numbers need to decrease because the integration is bad, and the criminality has connections to migration. Löfven however, he brought proposals forward that would increase the migration.[200]

There was a factual issue that did not have to do with the government reshuffle to do. It was the prime minister with his other ministers that mentioned the factual issue. In conjunction with this *Liberalerna* threatened to leave if the sharpens the proposal about humanitarian protection basis. *Liberalerna* did not think that the original promises from the January agreement about migration has been fulfilled. Party leader for *Liberalerna* said that if they do not follow through with the promises, the party will cancel the January agreement and stop supporting the government.[201]

Stefan Löfven was then open with an extra election. The Attorney General Morgan Johansson said that the proposal is not a big thing and will not lead to more resident permits because it will only apply to persons with temporary resident permits. He says that the text need to become more understandable and that a government crisis and an eventual extra election is not necessary. The proposal was changed in an effort to stop *Liberalerna* from operate a government crisis.[202]

Miljöpartiet did not want the proposal that residence permits would primarily be temporary. *Miljöpartiet* supported 3 out of the 26 proposals while *Socialdemokraterna* supported all of them. *Miljöpartiet* and *Socialdemokraterna* compromised by sending all proposals for referral and sending in new proposals.[203]

Isabella Lövin said that persons without reason for protection would need to leave the country however the four that was represented spoke the opposite way:

- Persons that have been in Sweden for a long time with temporary residence permits and has established themselves, but the situation in the home country has improved can stay in Sweden
- Unaccompanied migrants that turn 18 years during their time in Sweden and that does not have protection reasons can stay Sweden

- The income support for the unaccompanied that has been rejected, but is covered by the college amnesty facilitates
- Quota refugees can also receive extended rights for relative immigration

It was these suggestions were contributing causes for the 2015 migrant crisis.[203]

In conjunction with *Miljöpartiet* wanting to leave the government for the asylum migration legislation, they also demanded that the oil refinery that *Preem* planned to expand were to be cancelled because of its carbon dioxide emissions. *Miljöpartiet* left the message that the government would say no to *Preem's* project. *Socialdemokraterna* secretly wanted the project to continue due to *Preem* readjust to fossil-free production and the job opportunities that would be created. The judgement about permission is at the hands of the government, however it is with the current legislation that the judgement is based upon otherwise the Supreme Administrative Court, or the EU court will reject it. Legal justification for stopping the oil refinery is missing; the stop-law can not be applied on the operation because it is included in the EU`s trade and emission rights.[199]

The third matter that leads *Miljöpartiet* towards leaving the government is the expansion of Arlanda. *Miljöpartiet* claimed that there was an agreement to stop the expansion of Arlanda. *Socialdemokraterna* demented the claim.[198]

In the January agreement that made the government, the change of the rules of order were a vital part of the agreement and it made it possible for *Centerpatiet* and *Liberalerna* to agree to the January agreement. The change would be that instead of it being two different reasons for a dismissal, there would be five of them and extending the right to dismiss someone because of personal reasons. *Vänsterpartiet* did not want this to happen, and they threatened Stefan Löfven by stating that they will release a declaration of mistrust if they change the legislation around labor law. If *Vänsterpartiet* releases the declaration of mistrust, the opposition will vote yes to discontinue the government.[204] The employer organization *Svenskt näringsliv* has advanced their positions regarding change in the rules of order and made changes themselves. Martin Klepke says that it is better with negotiations than with a government crisis.[205] Stefan Löfven hoped that the contributors of the labor market would solve this situation on their own because he is critical towards the suggestions that the investigation has recommended. *Centerpartiet* and *Liberlaerna* on the other hand wants the whole legislation to follow through.[204] *LO* could not solve the issue as Stefan Löfven wanted and it was up to the politicians to make negotiations about legislation. *Vänsterpartiet* wants the investigation to be thrown away while *Liberalerna* and *Centerpartiet* wants it to continue.[199] In the end *Vänsterpartiet* did not release the declaration of mistrust.

The Social democrats of Sweden was getting closer to a proposal of market rents for rental apartments.[206 00:00-00:17] Market rents means that landlords can freely set the price for the apartment.[207] The government consisted of *Socialdemokraterna, Miljöpartiet, Liberalerna and Centerpartiet* with support from *Vänsterpartiet* and the opposition consisted of *Moderaterna, Kristdemokraterna* and *Sverigedemokraterna*. It was *Vänsterpartiet* who threatened *Socialdemokraterna* with saying that if they proceed with market rents, they will release a declaration of mistrust.[206 00:00-00:17] A declaration of mistrust is voted for in the parliament and would mean that the government and the authorities will verify if the government has done their job well or not.[208] Even though *Vänsterpartiet* threatened with it, it was *Sverigedemokraterna* who went to the parliament with the declaration of mistrust.[206 00:00-00:17] The reason for the declaration of mistrust from *Sverigedemokraterna* was the long healthcare queue, the low pensions and the low safety due to the criminality.[206 00:20-00:25] *Vänsterpartiet* were ready to support *Sverigedemokraterna* and if no one would change their stance, the declaration of mistrust would go through.[206 00:40-00:47] *Vänsterpartiet* were to release the declaration and discontinue the government on Monday the 21st of June if they were to implement market rents.[209 00:09-00:16] Both the *Kristdemokraterna* and *Moderaterna* would vote with *Vänsterpartiet and Sverigedemokraterna* for the declaration of mistrust.[209 00:41-00:50] Even though *Socialdemokraterna* did not apply market rents, *Vänsterpartiet* made themselves ready along with *Moderaterna, Kristdemokraterna and Sverigedemokraterna* to discontinue the government[210 00:40-00:48] and they could do that because they had 182 mandates against 167. On the 21st of July the government was discontinued;[211 00:05-00:07] the government was discontinued and Stefan Löfven had to resign[211]

[00:05-00:08] and Stefan Löfven had two options, he would either resign as prime minister and give the mission to floor leader Andreas Norlén who would carry through floor leader rounds with the same distribution of seats or Löfven could choose to implement an extra election[212] [00:52-01:17] and he had a week to decide.[213] [00.12-00:17] Annie Lööf of *Centerpartiet* wanted to continue *januariavtalet* which is the agreement that formed the government. she was able to deny market rents because the parliament voted against it, however she is still supporting the idea.[214] [00:11-01:22] *Liberalerna* walked away from *januariavtalet*[215] [02:46-02:50] and joined the opposition. During this time *Socialdemokraterna* were still preparing for an extra election.[215] [00:05-00:08] On the 24th of June, Stefan Löfven said that he would resign and therefore the next government would be decided by floor leader rounds.[216] [00:06-00:14] Stefan Löfven(So) wanted his budget to be chosen if he would be chosen as prime minister, but he wanted to resign if his budget would not be voted forward.[217] [01:00-01:19] Before the prime ministerial vote, Stefan Löfven had the biggest support out of the two potential prime ministers, he had 175 mandates while the parti leader for *moderaterna* Ulf Kristersson(Mo) had 174[218] [00:36-00:45] the maverick Amineh Kakabaveh, *Vänsterpartiet*, *miljöpartiet* and *Centerpartiet* supported Löfven(So).[219] [02:28-02:48] In the final decision Stefan Löfven was voted for.[216] [00:10-00:17]

After Stefan Löfven(So) retired, Magdalen Andersson(So) became the prime minister. When she was voted for with a single vote margin.[220] [00:02-00:06] The thing that determined was that Amine Kakabaveh(-) voted Andersson(So) through.[220] [00:07-00:14] The vote from Kakabaveh was bought by *Socialdemokraterna*[220] [01:22-01:28] by the signing of an agreement between the two parts[220] [01:30-01:34] With the agreement *Socialdemokraterna* will initiate a deeper relationship with the Kurdish party *PYD*[220] [01:45-01:50] *PYD* are stamped as terrorists by *EU* and the US.[220] [02:16-02:18] Shortly thereafter the parliament voted through a budget from *Moderaterna*, *Kristdemokraterna*, and *Sverigedemokraterna*[221] [00:44-00:49] meaning that their budget will be utilised by the current government until the election in September 2022.[221] [00:51-00:59] *Miljöpartiet* said that they did not want to support a budget from the right parties,[222] [00:11-00:17] and they threatened to leave the government.[222] [00:01-00:06] Jimmie Åkesson(Sd) said that if Per Bolund(Mp) is included in the government, he then will send in a declaration of mistrust.[223] [01:13-01:21] Annie Lööf(C) is included in the government with the left parties while she voted through a budget from the right parties because she did not want to vote through a budget from the left because *Vänsterpartiet* helped to set it up.[223] [02:27-02:39] *Miljöpartiet* left the government because of the budget.[224] [00:32-00:36] Magdalena Andersson(So) resigned as a prime minster after seven hours[225] [0:08-00:14] She was later chosen to a prime minister again.[226] [00:22-00:26]

4.6 Covid-19 Statistics

Sweden reporting of deaths is not up to date due to *Folkhälsomyndigheten* not reporting all deaths at the exact date of its occurrence. The delay of the reporting of a death can be up to a month. Most of the delayed deaths are reported five to 14 days after its occurrence.[227] The statsistics has been swayed in the other direction as well for example in the region of Uppsala, patients who are hospitalised for other reasons than Covid-19 are tested for it and if it comes out positive; they are counted as a Covid-19 patient. The fact that they have Covid-19 is important, however they should not be counted as hospitalised for Covid-19 unless they are treated for Covid-19 aswell as their initial reason for seeeking hospital care.[228] The reason for why Sweden´s statistics are deceptive Is because Sweden reports their cases based upon their time of death, Ourworldinadata reports their deaths based on date of report; it ends up with Sweden reporting deaths for several days on a single day and Ourworldindata reporting the Swedish deaths based upon the day of report.[227] For the 25th of March 2020 the deaths were at 42 people, but after three revisions, the number of deaths went up to 373.[230]

An investigation done by *TT* in April 2020 showed that *Folkhälsomyndigheten* was slow to report the amount of Covid deaths. After revisions from *TT* the death toll doubled.[230] In October 2020 Sweden´s corona deaths were not registered to *ECDC* correctly because the deaths was not registered the same day as they were instead you will have to wait a couple of days for the correct number of deaths.[229] The delay to see the actual death toll could go up towards two weeks. The most amount of delay was during April to July 2020 and November 2020 and May 2021.[227]

4.7 "We are just like any other country"

The goverent at the time of the Covid-19 pandemic waned to push a good Sweden image and tegnelll was on it. He worked both domestically and foreignally. As mentioned earlier Tegnell said that we could be rid of the virus during the summer of 2020 and therefore he was comfortable with not wanting to worry the public fore the Autumn 2020.

The elderly people is a risk group for Covid-19 and given the complications of the elderly care as well as the low pensions; they were at great risk of being infected.

The government let *Folkhälsomyndigheten* do most of the work regarding policies. The government were more a passive. Given that Sweden has three different governing bodies, it makes it easy for the politicians to blame eachother. The political tension between the left and the right parties only resulted in political disagreements. The parties were more concerned in other political areas than Covid-19 during the crisis.

5. Corona

A theme in the Swedish strategy has been that Tegnell does not want to put in measures where you do not know what the effect will be. Meaning he does not want to set in measures with theoretical effects[231] for example Annie Lööf(C) suggested that we should lockdown shopping centers and department stores, but Tegnell said that we do not know what effect that it has epidemiologically, but that it has bad societal effects.[232]

5.1 Testing

Dr Tedros Adhanom Ghebreyesus had a message for all countries to test persons,[130 17:08-17:21] however Sweden has had a lot of problems with testing according to Anders Tegnell, but not according to others. Tegnell said that "We know there is countries that has tested a lot like Germany for example that now anyway have gone very problematic situation with rising cases and fast death toll"[130 16:32-16:41 Translated quote] because he does not understand that testing does not have to do with the amount of people who dies and does not understand that when you test people for Covid-19 the amount of cases of Covid-19 will rise because people are infected by it. On the twelfth of March

2020 Tegnell said that with the number of cases, tracing and testing would not be viable and that it would not stop the epidemic.[130 08:35-08:44] Two days later Tegnell announced that they would stop the testing.[130 08:44-08:50] The reason Tegnells gives for the low testing in the beginning of the pandemic is that resources were low and it was only people who came to the health care and a small amount people in the elderly care that could be tested.[130 09:10-09:54] and Tegnell has said that they tested as much as possible with the resources that they possessed[130 10:07-10:21] and they have used their resources as critically as possible.[130 11:10-11:20] Tegnell said that it was not necessary to test people when Sweden came into a pandemic phase because the test needs to be followed-up and Sweden did not have such resources and therefore the tests became useless in his opinion. He thinks that the measures around is the things that matters which needed a lot of resources which were not there,[130 11:50-12:30] he also says that when you test someone, you have to give the person good advice to the person that tested positive and also tracing around the person.[130 18:24-18:40] The scientist and professor Harriete Whallberg said that the low testing was not as a result of a shortage of resources, it was that *Folkhälsomyndigheten* did not talk to the government about testing and tracing.[130 13:30-13:49] The systemic problems around tracing was that it took time to connect the private university laboratories to the health care[130 14:00-14:27] and the region does everything by themselves and they needed resources from academic and private actors. The regions needed to reset so that they could handle social security numbers and provide patient safety.[130 15:06-15:30]

	PCR-tests	Antibody tests
Tests in total	15 564 640	1 715 269
Tests per capita	1,49959	0,165259
Tests per 1 000	15 564,6	1 715,2
Tests per 1 000 000	15,6	1,7

The tests per 1 000 000 and tests per 1 000 is rounded to one decimal. The tests per capita is calculated with the amount of people living in Sweden being 10 379 295. It is rounded to five decimals. The amount of tests is based upon numbers from *Fokhälsomyndigheten* and the amount of tests done in 2020 and 2021.

5.2 Tegnell on facial masks

Despite that Tedros Adhanom Ghebreyesus recommended governments to encourage the public to wear masks wear it is difficult with social distancing on the 5th of June 2020,[187 43:03-43:17], the only place it has been is during rushing hours in public transport early 2021.[130 19:53-19:57] Tegnell does not think that facial masks make any significant difference with the spread of infection and therefore has not put out any measures regarding the facial masks.[187 42:36-42-44] *Folkhälsomyndigheten* has said that facial masks are not needed in normal situations and that distance is enough.[233]

Folkhälsomyndigheten recommended the hospital of Sahlgrenska to not wear face masks around infected patients. The protective equipment that they were obligated to use were face shield or a combination of protective glasses and liquid repellent face masks. The staff is still recommended to wear face masks or respiratory protection in situation with higher risk of infection and the staff is split about using face masks. Director of health and medical care in Västra Götaland Ann Söderström said that the early recommendations was too strict and that she trusts the care hygienist to recommend proper protective equipment. She thinks that *Fokhälsomyndigheten* will change recommendations for the whole country. The initiative was inspired by *WHO*. From a chart Söderström she interpreted that you would not need facial masks and a face shield at the same time.[234] Sweden´s regions and municipalities does not demand face masks to be worn in situations where staff is close to patients. The decision of wearing face masks are to be determined from the situation instead.[170] When other countries demanded face masks on flights, Sweden did not follow through and does not recommend it either because the guidelines says that face masks are not needed in everyday life.[235]

When companies started to produce protective equipment for the healthcare late March 2020 *Arbetsmiljöverket* did not approve of it because the equipment even though the EU commission has came out and said that in crisis the healthcare staff can wear equipment that is not approved, however it only applies when *Socialstyrelsen* or *MSB*, the authority for societal protection, approve of protective equipment and thereafter distributes it.[236] During this period only Malmö and Lund, the staff needed 1 000 face shields a day. The region of Skåne found a way to go around the legislation via the region being the head of the production while having a collaboration with persons and companies that produces.[237] Attendo introduced facial masks for their domestic service staff and reduced the spread of infection by 96%, but they had to brake the law to save lives as the facial masks that were utilised were not CE marked which violates the law.[238]

5.3 Denying herd immunity strategy

When Tegnell reacted to old videos of him speaking about the Swedish herd immunity strategy he responded with saying that the more immune people there is, the bigger the braking effect you will have.[130 32:57-33:05] Even though it is true, it should not have more of an effect or even a significant effect in comparison to the other measures the state puts in. He said that immunity played a small role in their models[130 34:10-34:24] and that every single country has it in their models.[130 33:48-34:03] He thinks that it plays a role in the strategy and that it makes it easier to keep track of other measures.[130 35:05-35:14]

In the middle of March 2020 Tegnell said that reaching herd immunity through enough people being infected was not the motive, however it was something that was likely to happen. Annika Linde perceived that reaching natural herd immunity was the motive with the strategy that *Folkhälsomyndigheten* developed.[239] In April Tegnell predicted that Stockholm would be among the first places that develops herd immunity and predicted it to be reached in May 2020. Tegnell said that their data output is only as good as the data input and that ""We will see if they are right"".[163-164] The Swedish ambassador in Washington Karin Ulrika Olofsdotter said that 30 percent of people in Stockholm had reached a level of immunity and that Stockholm would reach herd immunity in May repeating what Tegnell said.[240]

An infection control physician Anders Nystedt said that Sweden´s strategy was to slowly gain a natural immunity.[133] [00:10-00:20] Nystedt predicted that the immunity would be 10 percent in Norrbotten, but it turned out to be 2 percent in June. When *Folkhälsomyndigheten* was asked whether immunity was a regional goal for Norrbotten or a national goal. They said that it was both, but primarily the motive of *Folkhälsomyndigheten*.[133]

5.4 Schools

There are no effects regarding closing schools in pandemic according to Tegnell in late February 2020. It would rather lead to worse effects since people would meet other persons in other contexts instead according to Tegnell.[109]

During the Spring 2020 children could be leaved at kindergarten if they had been symptom free, but during Autumn, parent could leave their children if they left them after seven days of mild symptoms or after two days free from symptoms.[241] There are witnesses for when staff in kindergartens sends children home to their parents, they are scolded. Principals are supporting the parents and legitimises that children with symptoms stays in the kindergarten.[242] When *SIFO* made a survey 6 out of 10 kindergarten teachers had been in a situation where they had been in a conflict with a parent leaving their child with symptoms.[241] During a *Folkhälsomyndigheten* allowed corona stricken parents to leave their children at kindergarten. When *Folkhälsomyndigheten* changed it so that the parents could not, it was because of the sake of the children not because of the risk of spreading it further.[243]

Elementary schools were held opened for the most part and if the students in elementary school did not come to school because of worried parents, the parents were reported to social services and received fines.[244] When Swedish school children returned to class after Summer 2020, parents and experts said that there should be more responsible policies such as mask wearing mandatorily, however given Tegnells attitude towards masks; masks did not become mandatory. There have been scientific studies from countries South Korea, the US, Israel and Sweden that says that it is clear that school-age children spreads the virus to a wider group of people. The professor of microbial pathogenesis Cecilia Söderberg-Nauclér however said that there was not any knowledge about the spread of infection in schools.[247]
Folkhälsomyndigheten had traced the infections in schools for a long time but was established that high school students stood for 20 percent of the infections. *Folkhälsomyndigheten* decided to stop with the tracing of infections after week 49 2020.[245]

Even though Tegnell claimed that they tried to find a strategy which does not involve the closing of schools,[130 06:24-06:51] the government shifted to distance education for college schools in March 2020[246] and it was a result of *Folhälsomyndigheten* recommending it. This was also the first big measure that Sweden did. Colleges and universities had distance education from March 2020 however elementary schools had distance from May 2020. For the autumn term after the summer break colleges went to 20% distance education meaning that students would be at home one day of the week and that was kept until right before the Christmas break where the colleges went to 100% distance education. The measures taken for the schools only worsened the situation for the students because they were taken only days before they were introduced.

5.5 Sweden ruining it for other countries

When a corona case came up in Österbotten, it was established that the person was infected from a trip to Sweden. A Finnish doctor said that every corona case from there could be traced back to Sweden.[248]Tegnel tried to affect Finland´s Covid-strategy wanting them to adopt a less strict strategy.

Giesecke went on Norwegian media to convince the Norwegians of Sweden´s herd immunity strategy being superior to Norway´s strategy because Sweden would reach herd immunity in May 2020 while Norway would have the same death toll as other countries. He wrote to Preben Aavitsland to repeat the same message to the Norwegian Institute of Public Helath.[249]

Tegnell was qouted in an article in *The Times of India* about how a vaccine was far off. The Indian political party Swarna Bharat Party was in support of Tegnells ideas of a herd immunity strategy. Tegnell preached to India that having children in school was not going to affect the spread of infection. In an interview Giesecke told Rahul Gandhi of India that everyone in the world will be infected and 99 percent of infected people will have few symptoms or no symptoms. Giesecke recommended India not to have a lockdown because the economy will suffer and to protect the frail and elderly and ""let the other people have the infection"". He told Gandhi that a severe lockdown might lead to more deaths than corona itself.[249]

Boris Johnson were in a number of Zoom calls for advice to decide the next steps. Tegnell was there and told him to reject a second lockdown.[249]

Giesecke went to the Irish Oireachtas Committee and presented the herd immunity strategy to convince the Irishmen to imlplement it. He was heavily refuted.[249]

Tegnell went to Brazil with Johanna Brismar-Skoog to present how Sweden has combatted the pandemic. They presented Sweden´s strategy as succesful and lied aswell as hid drawbacks. They told Brazil everyone got the same amount of hospital care, andthe decision to keep schools open was good. He spoke badly of lockdowns and facial masks. They did not mention that testing was limited. Tegnell told them herd immunity were slowing down the spread of the virus and that there had not been reinfections. After following Sweden´s example, Brazil recorded 666 000 deaths.[249]

During the summer of 2020 a lot of countries gave Swedes travel bans despite Tegnell´s claims about the Swedes being immune enough to travel. Denmark only welcomes Swedes with a couple of demands: Swedes are only welcome if they have a cottage, family or partner in Denmark or if Denmark is a transit destination. Greece made randomized testing if the traveller comes from an airport with high risk of infection and Arlanda is one of those airports. Malta did not allow Swedes. The Czech Republic allows Swedes, but Swedes are on top of the list of spread of infection. Holland allowed Swedes, but Swedes are one of multiple nationalities that had to be in a two-week quarantine. Swedes were not welcome in the Baltic States.[250] The Swedish minister of foreign affairs Anne Linde thought that it was discriminating that Cypress is not allowing Swedes there when they are allowing Danes and Norwegians as tourists.[157-158] Tegnell thinks that Swedes should be welcome like other people. He says that open borders are always good and that closed borders are a bad idea.[113] Tegnell tried to affect the rest of Europe when he wrote a letter to the *ECDC* and warned them about recommending masks because it would spread panic and also indicate that the coronavirus is airborne. He has said that the idea that the attitude towards masks being silver bullets are dangerous and the evidence for facial masks are weak.[108] Tegnell was in a meeting the 17th of Sepember regarding Great Britain´s decision for a lockdown. Tegnell amongst other were described as proponent of a "herd immunity" approach.[251]

5.6 Covid healthcare

The hospital of Salhgrenska was supposed to be free from corona patients.[20] They decided to use a field hospital for the corona patients. There are intensive care places that are empty as a result of not being used for corona patients.[21] In the field hospital in Göteborg doctors said that there is no water or drains, the patients are located closer to each other than in normal departments. The ventilations are bad and the respirators are outdated.[22] Every corona patient is not taken care of in the field hospital, the most seriously ill are taken care of inside the hospital.[23] A doctor said that the hospital care in the field hospital is not the best intensive care that could be given.[24] The operations manager Henrik Sundman said that the hospital care in the field hospital is of the same quality as in the hospital and that he sees it develop further.[25] After critique of the field hospital, it was decided that the corona patients would be taken care of inside the hospital.[26]

In a room with eight patients there needed to be three teams with each containing: a team responsible intensive care nurse, two anaesthesia or intensive care nurses, two assistant nurses or surgical nurses and three intensive care physicians. The lack of staff makes it so that the staff need to take fluid replacement.[252] In 2020 99% of the intensive care beds were filled mid-December. There was a lack of staff and Sweden needed help from other countries.[253] It was not the only time Sweden needed help with staff because in late May the general lack of staff for thbergste intensive care made Sweden request staff from other countries for the second time. The municipalities and regions of Sweden asked for intensive care staff from the Nordic countries and Norway and Denmark gave them green light. Sweden has had lack of specialist nurse for 15 years and the resources for it has been there, but the planning has not.[254] For a third time 16 out of 21 of Swedens regions needed more staff from the Nordic countries in October.[255] Nursing homes, hospitals and hospital staff did not have masks early in the pandemic because it was a product with a price and the government did not make protective equipment a priority,[256 15:37-15:59] even though it was known that mouth covers were effective.[256 16:59-17-14]

There are two main groups that comes to the intensive care. The first group comes from the intensive care and has become very ill at home which is either caused by Covid or that they have Covid and bacteria in their lungs. The second group has received treatment with high-flow oxygen at the infection clinic, but it does not work properly. They come after a few days and sometimes the treatment with high-flow oxygen is continued, but often they need to be intubated and receive respiratory care. All the vital parameters are checked on the patients such as pulse and blood pressure, respiration and oxygenation of the blood all the time. The patients have constantly a tube that are in an artery so that blood can be drawn at any time without pricking the patient for a blood test. It is mostly used to know how the breathing works. The urine production is checked every hour. When the body of the patient's body can not cleanse the blood by itself, the patient receives dialysis.[252]

The Covid patients receives multiple medicines. It is medicines used for other intensive care patients, but some medicines are given in higher dosages for example cortisone to dampen inflammation and blood thinning agents to avoid blood clots in lungs, and other organs which is used early. Some medicines are given with pumps so that the patient receives the right dose at the right time at the right velocity. Anticoagulants are used early. The patients produce a lot of thick mucus after three to four days and it needs to be dealt with immediately before airway obstruction occurs. It is dealt with by suck it clean via bronchoscopy.[252]

In the first week, they need to be put to sleep deeper with respirator, it often requires muscle relaxants so that the breathing can be taken over with the respirator and the way of the breath can be determined by the staff. When the lungs and the body has started to recover, it is time to wake the patient up again and slowly phase the respirator out. It becomes a period of coughing and irritation in the lungs, and it is hard to wake the patient. When they receive respirator care, it becomes an elongated process, or they have to be put to sleep and the breathing becomes controlled by the staff. The inflammation runs amok in the body due to the viral disease which leads to small clots in several organs, and mainly affects the lungs with a very special lung injury as a result.[252]

During Spring 2020 almost all patients had kidney failure, but at the end of 2020, there was only a few. There were some patients with severe heart failure, but the staff has learned more and more about fluid treatment. The patient was anxious during the Spring of 2020 which was a result of them being sicker in the beginning because of the premises and the staff is better adapted to the disease.[252]

Jon Tallinger is a whistleblower who exposed the deficiencies in the healthcare that the politicians are behind in May 2020. Tallinger received a video instruction from the region where they instructed that everyone should care plan their elderly patients. Care planning means that one should take a decision if the patient receives care or not. The instruction video instructed doctors to treat patients palliatively with morphine when they have dyspnea. Oxygen was not mentioned.[256 01:35-01:21] The problem that Tallinger mentions that if the patient is treated via palliative care with morphine and there is no oxygen, and the patient is not sent to the hospital; the patient will suffocate, and their anxiety is taken away because there is no oxygen in elderly homes.[02:51-03:14] He received a document from the region that explained that elderly with risk factors should not be taken to the hospital.[256 04:04-04-11] There are some that says that oxygen is a problem in terms of skill and availability, but according to Tallinger it does not take any skill to administer oxygen,[256 07:39-07:44] even though it is established that only educated personnel at hospitals can handle oxygen.[257] Sweden has an abundance of oxygen because there are factories for oxygen.[256 19:30-19:41] There are some that says that COPD is a reason not to give a patient oxygen and it is better to let them die of carbon dioxide and narcosis than it is letting them die of morphine.[256] 06:50-09:20

The patients get their teeth brushed in the morning and in the evening and at lunch they receive mouth wash with bactericidal to reduce the risk of bacteria going down the airways and causing bacterial pneumonia. During the initial days, the patient lies on the belly as much as possible and it was extraordinarily successful for the Covid-patients in the intensive care. The patients´ positions are changed at least every third hour to reduce risk of pressure ulcers and some areas of the body are sensitive meaning a lot of pillows are used. The patient receives physiotherapy to keep their joints mobile. When the patient has woken up, their lungs are trained. They can breathe a few minutes the first time and then it improves for every day until they can breathe by themselves.[258]

The protective medical equipment that are required for working at the Covid intensive care is plastic apron, face shield, respiratory protection and a respiratory protection. When the staff leaves the section, they must take hand sanitizer.[258] Sweden had 7 300 000 face masks that was bought between 1969 and 1994. They cost 75 Swedish crowns a piece. In total it was about 547 500 000 Swedish crowns. They were burnt in the beginning of 2000. The destruction of them cost between 10 950 000 and 14 600 000 Swedish crowns in total.[258] The former minister of the interior affairs Anders Ygeman(So) said in 2017 that we should ""forget stocks of face masks, provisions and other necessities"".[259] As soon as by the 25th of March 2020, healthcare staff said that their protective equipment would last two to three days forward. While the stash of equipment was low, regions loosened their rules of equipment by not demanding that staff has long sleeve clothes.[260] Initially the amount of medical equipment was low enough for Gröna Lund to sent their rain coats as protective equipment. *Socialstyrelsen* said that they gave enough protection and sent ten at first. On the first of April 2020, they sent 10 000 of them.[262] *Folkhälsomyndigheten* and the regions lowered the requirements for protective equipment by not requiring facial masks and long sleeved protective clothing, it was not because they were not needed even though they motivated their choice by stating that they have new information about Covid-19, it was rather due to lack of protective equipment.[261]

5.7 Prioritisations in the healthcare

Aftonbladet took part of a document where it was revealed that persons with the biological age of 80 and over, biological age of 70 to 80 that has a maximum of two organ failures, biological age of 60 to 70 that has a maximum of two organ failures would not receive intensive care at Karolinska universitetsjukhuset and when the healthcare places are low.[263] *Socialstyrelsen* sent out a document where it said that people who are able to do household chores would be prioritised. The elderly would not receive care unless they had an operation. It would be applied when the healthcare places are short, but they were already in place in May 2020 when the document came out. It was not applied all over the country though.[264] It is not surprising that it is the elderly that is victims to this since the former Social minister Annika Strandhäll(So) said that the muslim migration is not a problem for the healthcare, it is rather the elderly that is a problem for the healthcare.[265] An 81-year-old at a retirement home received corona, but instead of being sent to the hospital, he received morphine. When his son demanded that he would be treated with nutrition, he started to recover.[266] The prioritisations are put in place due to low staff in the hospitals,[267] premises and equipment.[180] A 96-year-old at a retirement home had corona symptoms, but she was denied a corona test. There was no oxygen there.[268] A daughter came to her mother who is 97 years old in a retirement home because she had corona symptoms. When the daughter asked why she was not sent to the hospital, she was told that her mother was too old. It stood that the mother received palliative care, but the only thing the mother was offered was paracetamol and an open window. Her oxygenation was at 60%, but she did not receive oxygenation treatment. The mother probably died because of corona, but she did not get tested.[269]

5.8 Tegnell on Lockdown

The reason for the anti-lockdown strategy is the attitude towards it. Tegnell thinks that it does not have an effect and that is does not help during longer periods. He says that the negative effect is that it will put more pressure on the healthcare because the curve on the infection graph will be steeper.[130 23:26-23:53] He says that the countries that has had strict lockdowns has had higher death tolls and the cost of a lockdown is too much.[130 24:35-24:57]

A lockdown is not in question because Tegnell is saying that Sweden already has a shutdown.[130 27:38-28:13] Stefan Löfven said that Sweden had underestimated the virus during the last period of 2020 and the intensive-care units in Stockholm became overwhelmed. In November 2020, they recorded 8088 deaths which has only been beaten by Sweden´s worst month of the H1N1-influenza pandemic.[270] Despite the result from November Stefan Löfven chose to change the measures against corona, but the measures were not restrictive enough, it was a recommendation against gatherings consisting of more than 8 people.[271] Tegnell has despite critics suggested Sweden´s approach is better than strict lockdowns when it comes to being equipped for the next coming wave.[253]

5.9 The data does not back Anders Tegnell

Whenever Anders Tegnell has critisized something, he has said that the data does not support it, however after the two first years of the Covid-19 pandemic, Sweden only tested the amount of people equivalent to one and a half of the whole polpulation. The biggest numbers of Covid cases were observed in January 2022 when everyone could get their first two jabs of vaccine.

This shows that Sweden needed way more testing than they had due to the fact that Sweden took an open society approach for their strategy. That is if the vaccines even were effective.

With the open society approach, one would think that facial masks are the key to the strategy succeding, however Tegnell has talked against them. He sees them as uneccesary and therefore they have not been recommended in public. The only exception is that they were recommended in public transport during rush hours, however the constant criticism against these made the public not want to wear them; even when they were recommended in public transport in all situations, people did not use them.

The herd immunity strategy that Anders Tegnell crafted with Tom Britton was only current while they were hopeful it was going to work. The goal was gong to be reached for the first summer in the summer of 2020, but it was not reached. The numbers on immunity were far lower than expected when they were measured. The strategy to save face was to simply deny that reaching herd immunity without a vaccine was the motive for the strategy.

Schools closed one after another when cases were revealed. The gymnasium school were closed at first in the middle of march 2020, but for some reason during the next term students were only at home for 20 percent of the time meaning one day a week. It just shows that *Folkhälsomyndigheten* did not really have a clue what to do. Holding a school totally closed and having distance education makes sence from a pandemic strategy perspective, but the decision to have 20 percent of the education at home were totally useless since the rest of the week is enough time for students to infect eachother.

Anders Tegnell and Johan Giesecke did not hold back on trying to influence other countris strategies. It was not only neighbours or European countries. It should not surprise anyone as Sweden has a superiority complex. While Swedes are not really nationalistic about their culture and history etcetera, politicians and political figures wants to apply Swedish standards in other countries. Swedes also affected other countries only by Sweden having as many infections as it had hence why Swedes were banned to travel more than other nationalities.

The healthcare was already suffering due to lack of financing, too much paperwork for the healthcare staff and bad staffing solutions among other things. Since gaslighting around facial masks, steps to avoid meeting people, the infectivity of corona and infectivity before symptoms were not enough. The last step in the process to indirectly kill people with the virus is to worsen the covid healthcare. Doctors were told to give people morphine instead of oxygen to treat patients and that is if they were said to have corona. A lot of elderly people at elderly homes were not tested before dying and therefore they died of Corona, but these cases were not counted as corona deaths.

6.1 Vaccine

In April Tegnell claimed that Sweden would gain an immunity before receiving the vaccine, but four months later in August he said that an immunity only reduces the spread and not that it completely stops the spread,[133] however the vaccinations still came in January 2021 and it was persons who lives in special accommodations for elderly or has home care, staff in the elderly care, health care and other sort of care that works close to these persons and persons who are in close contact with the said groups of persons who was prioritised in the first phase. In the second phase 65+ year olds, persons that has done bone marrow transplants or other organ transplant and their household contacts, persons with dialysis treatment and their household contacts, persons of the age of 18 and over that receives services because of disabilities, persons of the age of 18 and over that receives assistance allowance and staff that works close to the mentioned persons could vaccinate themselves. For the third phase persons between the ages of 60 and 64, pregnant woman that is over the age of 35 or has a BMI over 30 and persons between the ages of 18 and 59 that has a disease or condition that makes them more vulnerable to Covid-19 such as dementia, cognitive disabilities or psychological disability, persons that finds themselves in socially vulnerable situations, persons with chronic cardiovascular disease, including stroke and hypertension, chronic lung disease such as COPD and severe and unstable asthma, other conditions that lead to impaired lung function or impaired cough and secretion stagnation for example extreme obesity, neuromuscular diseases or multiple disabilities, chronic liver, kidney failure, diabetes type 1 and 2, conditions that involve severely weakened immune systems due to an illness or treatment and downs syndrome. In the fourth phase can persons in the ages of 18 to 59 vaccinate themselves. The persons that should be prioritised no matter phase is older people and persons with worse socioeconomic status.[272]

A lot of people that has not belonged to the valid prioritisation group has booked time for vaccinations.[273] They have sacrificed the elderly in special accommodations.[274 00:30-00:35] People uses different apps and webb boking to penetrate the vaccination queues and has to claim that they are another person. It is the same as forgery which can lead to up to six years in prison.[275] For example has 50 year olds outside of risk groups booked time for vaccination.[276] Care managers has penetrated the vaccination queues.[274] 00:00-00:03 The care managers were allowed the second dose when it was time for it. The care managers´ family members received vaccinations as well. This has led to different consequences elsewhere for example the Spanish minister of defence had to leave his position and a casino millionaire claiming to be a motel staff was arrested for trying to penetrate the vaccination queues.[277] During early February 2021 the vaccination scandal regarding people taking the vaccine when it is not their turn has happened in nine out of 21 regions.[278] Because of people penetrating the vaccination queue, the health centers has removed the option for people to book vaccination via the web.[279]

6.2 Breaktrough cases and the end of the pandemic

Brook Jackson revealed from witnesses that a subcontractor of Pfizer committed research fraud in phase iii. The company falsified data, unblinded, hired insufficiently educated vaccinators and was slow to follow up side-effects that was reported.[89]

In Israel there were reports of 60 percent of the hospitalized covid-patients were fully vaccinated. It is not only elderly patients; one of them is below the age of 40 and 16 between the age of 40 and 65.[280] Sir Patrick Vallance reported that 60 percent of the Covid-patients are vaccinated,[281] 15 percent are double vaccinated[282] and the remaining 25 percent has had a dose of vaccine. In Wales, the breakthrough rate, the proportion of people that received Corona after being vaccinated, was 96 percent and the median age was 37.[283] Age, long-term conditions such as asthma, diabetes or heart disease does not affect the chances of developing Covid after having two doses of vaccines, however people who are overweight or obese, poorer, and people with health conditions seems to be more likely to be infected by Covid. On the other hand, vaccinated people have fewer symptoms over a shorter period. The vaccinated people reports that they have headache, runny nose, sneezing, sore throat and loss of smell as symptoms.[282] The effectiveness of the Pfizer vaccine after the delta variant dropped to 50 percent for the elderly and 80 percent for the general population. Some health experts has said that the data that this is built on is problematic because some people over the age of 60 who appear unvaccinated are dead, the number of unvaccinated people who tests are not at a desirable rate, the number of people who are in decline of getting vaccinated also do not test themselves and people are deemed as severely ill when they do not receive proper health care is.[284] In Sweden more and more elderly began to get ill. From the 10th of August, the elderly began to become infected with Covid.

Folkhälsomyndigheten said that it was okay for persons with reduced immune system to receive a third dose during Autumn 2021 and then eventually in 2022 people in risk groups and people over the age of 80 would receive a third dose. The European Medicines Agency says that "fully vaccinated" people does not have a reason to receive a third dosage. The amount of vaccines were not a problem in this situation because *Doktor24* had to throw away 16 000 vaccines because the demand was low.[285] The people that could receive a third dose as of late October 2021 was: People born in 1956 or earlier, people who live in special accommodation for elders, people who receive home care or home health care, people who work at special accommodation for elders, the home health care service and home care service and people with reduced immune system due to illness or treatment and has permission from their doctor.[286] Even though news about breakthrough cases came in late August 2021

Folkhälsomyndigheten delayed with testing the double vaccinated until the 22nd of November.[287]

After the reports of breakthrough cases abroad in August, the parliament voted through vaccine passes. In the beginning of September 7 out 8 of the parliament parties was positive towards introducing vaccine passes after the first reports of breakthrough cases. The vaccine passes are there for operations to open for vaccinated people despite ongoing restrictions. Only one party says "No" and three says "Yes". The problem with their response is that they did not have the spread of infection in mind when considering their stance the problem was that ""it would mean an increased administration and it would be difficult to implement on a integrity secure way"". [Translated qoute][288] The remaining parties either says "maybe" or they have not finalised their stance. *Liberalerna* says that it is better if the power is in the hands of the companies and that it would mean that fragile people would be safer and therefore said "Yes". *Socialdemokraterna* had a national vaccine pass in mind since a time before. They say that it would be implemented with big events and that with the support of the corona law, there would be demands of vaccination for some operations. *Centerpartiet* can consider having vaccine passes for bigger events. *Moderaterna* wants the passes to ensure a successive regression to normal life for double vaccinated people. *Kristdemokraterna* wants passes to apply to big events. *Miljöpartiet* and *Sverigedemokraterna* did not have a stance.[288] It is not out of character that Sweden allowed vaccine passes because four months prior to that in May Sweden was the first country to introduce the green card of the EU that allows vaccinated people to travel in the EU.[289] 81 percent of Swedes wanted covid passes for concerts and other live events.[290]

The vaccines quite clearly did not do their part as in one day on the 26th of Janaury 2022, 40 055 covid cases was reported. That number is high conisdering the low amount of tests Sweden does. Both Tom Britton and Joakim Dillner predicted that Covid-19 would be over after the Omicron waves would start to weaken because of a global immunity. It was back in January that they predicted it,[291] however *Folkhälsomyndigheten* recommended a fifth vaccine dose at the start of the 2022 Autumn season for people in the ages 65 and over aswell as people in risk groups.[292] The term "fully vaccinated" loses its meaning when you hear that a fully vaccinated person who also is boosted caught Covid-19 twice with a 20 days inbetween the infections.[293]

The reason for the alleviation of Swedish restrictions is that the spread of infection has been decreased. From the first of June the following:

- The recommendation that one should only be with your nearest relatives is drawn back
- 3000 people are allowed at outdoor events
- 300 at indoor events, 50 people are allowed at private events
- 1800 people are allowed at demonstrations
- The recommendation to shop alone is drawn back
- Opening hours are free for restaurants and there is no limitation for the amount of people at outdoor servings
- 900 participants are allowed at exercise runs and contests recommendations about sporting alone is drawn back
- Associations are not recommended to not have meetings
- The recommendation about having face masks in public transport is taken away[294]
- In cinemas, theatres, and other events with seating indoors, 50 persons are allowed
- In sport-, culture- and other events outdoors with a standing audience, 100 persons are allowed
- In sport-, culture- and other events outdoors with a sitting audience, 500 persons are allowed

- Exercise races and competitions such as orienteering, sailing and cycling, 150 persons are allowed
- For flea- and other markets the rule about eight persons at public events does not apply
- For the amusement parks *Liseberg*, *Gröna Lund*, *Skara sommarland* and other permanent amusement parks, one person per 20 square meters are allowed
- Bars and taverns are allowed to serve alcohol until 10 pm and be open until 10:30 pm
- Summer camps and other activities for children are allowed
- Smaller cups and contests for children inside and outside are allowed

From the first of July:

- The limit for participants for public gatherings and public events indoors are increased to 50 persons and if the participants are assigned a seat the limit is increased to 300 persons
- In arrangements outdoors without assigned seats, 600 persons are allowed
- For arrangements with seats the limit for the amount of persons are 3000 persons
- Exerciser uns can have 900 participants
- The maximum for private gatherings are increased from eight to 50
- The recommendation to only socialize with the nearest social sphere is removed
- The recommendation for associations to call of, postpone or have meetings at a distance is eased off
- Serving places are allowed to have open for longer and the rules for the maximum per company and distance between companies are removed for outdoor serving places
- It is allowed to serve food and drinks standing outside

From the middle of July:

- Passenger limits on long distance public transport with busses and trains are removed
- The municipality can decide to repeal visit ban on specified places
- The recommendation about face masks in public transport is removed
- The regulation of a certain amount of square meters per person in indoors and outdoors environment is removed

In the second to last stage:

- The participant limitation for public gatherings is removed
- Restrictions on private gatherings are removed
- The regulations on indoor restaurants are completely removed

In the last stage all other restrictions that has been put because of Covid-19 are removed.[295] As part of the election campaign for *Sverigedemokraterna* was on a sausage tour. Jimmie Åkesson(Sd) said that it was good that you could meet people and shake hands.[296] 00:56-01:02 It was the 13 October 2021.

A pandemic may be a complicated situation to be in as a government, however that does not mean that the ruling politicians should hand over the responsibility towards their respective public health authorities. Anders Tegnell gave way too many red flags early on, but Stefan Löfven(So) could not care less.

The political parties were not aware of the uselessness of the vaccine passes in autumn 2021 and it reflects their lack of interest for the pandemic strategy.

Scan this QR-code to get in contact

Scan this QR-code to read my blog

7.1.2 Jantelagen
1. En lång utläggning om Jantelagens för- och nackdelar. 2013, 25 juli [7/9-2022]. Frökendrivkraft.
https://frokendrivkraft.wordpress.com/2013/07/25/en-lang-utlaggning-om-jantelagens-for-och-nackdelar/

7.1.3 Folkhemmet
2. SO-Rummet. Steriliseringspolitiken i Sverige. 2022. [7/9-2022].
https://www.so-rummet.se/fakta-artiklar/steriliseringspolitiken-i-sverige#

7.2.1 Folkhemmet erstwhile

3. Balz, Dan. Sweden sterilized thousands of 'Useless' citizens for decades. The washington post [Internet]. August 29th [5/9-2021]; Available from: https://www.washingtonpost.com/archive/politics/1997/08/29/sweden-sterilized-thousands-of-useless-citizens-for-decades/3b9abaac-c2a6-4be9-9b77-a147f5dc841b/

4. Butler, D. Eugenics scandal reveals silence of Swedish scientists. Nature; 1997. 389; 9. [5/9-2021]. Available from https://doi.org/10.1038/37848

5. Flam, Aron. Det här är en svensk tiger. Stockholm: Samizdat publishing. 2019.

6. Stockholmskällan. Välfärd för alla? [Internet]. 2022 [28/6-2023]. Available from: https://stockholmskallan.stockholm.se/teman/stockholms-sociala-historia/valfard-for-alla/

7. Shaw, Laura; Kurbegovic, Erna. Sweden. [5/9-2021]. Available from: https://eugenicsarchive.ca/discover/tree/51c2742697b8940a54000009

8. Budnik, Ruslan. The Nazis Weren't The First, Sweden First Started Sterilising People Who Were Not "Aryan". War History Online [Internet]. 12th of January 2019 [5/9-2021]; Available from: https://www.warhistoryonline.com/instant-articles/compulsory-sterilization.html

9. Bas-Wohlert, Camille; AFP; Swedish transgendereds battle for forced sterilization payouts. The Local [Internet]. 27th February 2013 [6/9-2021]. Available from: https://www.thelocal.se/20130227/46426

7.2.2 Folkhemmet currently

10. Angry Foreigner. The Whistleblower Dr Forced To Leave Sweden - Jon Tallinger on Swedish Healthcare Crisis [video file]. 2020, 13th September [10/9-2022]. Available from: https://www.youtube.com/watch?v=g4EBPmEmZd4&list=PLo0ElGp48iyL dNWvNqDo1cl_sqzeM-zHa

11. Hadžialić, Aida; Alkurdi, Talla; Sjöström, Jens; Johansson, Robert. Sveriges rikaste region klarar inte av vården. Aftonbladet [Internet]. 22 augusti 2021. [18/10-2022]; https://www.aftonbladet.se/debatt/a/0Gvyd6/sveriges-rikaste-region-klarar-inte-av-varden

12. Lindmark, Simon. SÖS måste spara 79 miljoner kronor i personalkostnader. Sveriges Radio [Internet]. 16 juli 2021 [18/9-2021]. Available from: https://sverigesradio.se/artikel/prognos-sos-behover-spara-79-miljoner-kronor-i-personalkostnader

13. P4 Stockholm. Upprörd vårdkår efter besparingsbesked: Det sista vi behöver just nu. Sveriges radio [Internet]. 20 juli 2021 [18/9-2021]. Available from: https://sverigesradio.se/artikel/upprord-vardkar-efter-besparingsbesked-kommer-fa-katastrofala-konsekvenser

14. Olsson, Daniel. Sverige skänkte bort sina fältsjukhus – bara två kvar. Expressen [Internet]. 5 april 2020 [1/1 2022]. Available from: https://www.expressen.se/gt/qs/sverige-skankte-bort-sina-faltsjukhus-bara-tva-kvar/

15. The Local. Is the second wave overloading Sweden´s intensive care units?. The Local [Internet]. 11th decmber 2020 [510-2021]. Available from: https://www.thelocal.se/20201211/is-the-second-wave-overloading-swedens-intensive-care-units/

16. Nyqvist, Oskar; Sima, Lotta; SVT Datajournalistik. Vårdskulden från inställda operationer. Svt [Internet]. 25 januari 2022 [30/9-2022]. Available from: https://www.svt.se/datajournalistik/vardskulden-fran-installda-operationer/

17. Palm, Fanny. Långa operationsköer gör att tarmcancer inte går att bota. SVT [Internet]. 24 januari 2018 [27/8-2021]. Available from: https://www.svt.se/nyheter/lokalt/skane/lakare-pa-sus-slar-larm-langa-operationskoer-gor-att-cancer-inte-gar-att-bota

18. Awad, Akil, Hildebrand, Karin. "Orimligt att sjukvården ständigt måste skyddas". Svenska Dagbladet [Internet]. 14 januari 2022 [28/9-2022]. Available from: https://www.svd.se/a/k61aBk/awad-och-hildebrand-orimligt-att-sjukvarden-standigt-maste-skyddas

19. Boström, Håkan. Håkan Boström: Hur Sverige slarvade bort sin beredskap. Göteborgsposten [Internet]. 30 mars 2020 [1/1-2022]. Available from: https://www.gp.se/ledare/hur-sverige-slarvade-bort-sin-beredskap-1.26107481

20. Björk, Frida. Nu öppnas IVA-platser för coronapatienter på Sahlgrenska. Svt [Internet]. 28 april 2020 [1/1-2022]. Available from: https://www.svt.se/nyheter/lokalt/vast/nu-oppnas-iva-platser-for-coronapatienter-pa-sahlgrenska

21. Björk, Frida. Överläkare slår larm om tältet på Östra: "Riskerar människors liv. Svt [Online]. 12 april 2020 [1/1-2022].Available from: https://www.svt.se/nyheter/lokalt/vast/overlakare-slar-larm-om-taltet-pa-ostra-riskerar-manniskors-liv

22. SVT Nyheter. Läkare slår larm om nya fältsjukhuset i Göteborg. [Internet]. 11 april 2020. [1/1-2022]. Available from: https://www.svt.se/nyheter/snabbkollen/lakare-slar-larm-om-nya-faltsjukhuset-i-goteborg

23. Rogsten, Eva. Läkarna slår larm – om fältsjukhuset. Expressen [Internet]. 12 april 2020 [1/1-2022]. Available from: https://www.expressen.se/gt/lakarna-slar-larm-om-faltsjukhuset/

24. Headtopics. Överläkare slår larm om tältet på Östra: "Riskerar människors liv". 11 april 2020 [1/1-2022]. Available from: https://headtopics.com/se/overlakare-sl-r-larm-om-taltet-p-ostra-riskerar-manniskors-liv-12389459

25. Bornman, Jens /TT. Fältsjukhuset i gång trots kritik. Dagens medicin [Internet]. 15 april 2020 [1/1-2022]. Available from: https://www.dagensmedicin.se/alla-nyheter/nyheter/faltsjukhuset-i-gang-trots-kritik/

26. Björk, Frida. Sahlgrenskas vändning: Stopp för nya patienter till fältsjukhuset. Svt [Internet]. 19 april 2020 [1/1-2022]. Available from: https://www.svt.se/nyheter/lokalt/vast/sahlgrenskas-beslut-stopp-for-patienter-till-faltsjukhuset

27. Askerup, Karin Matteson. Tusntals ringde 112 utan att få svar. Göteborgsposten [Internet]. 10 januari 2005 [15/8-2022]. Available from: https://www.gp.se/nyheter/sverige/tusentals-ringde-112-br-utan-att-f%C3%A5-svar-1.1216477

28. Blohm, Lisa. Kritiserad larmcentral får vara kvar. Dagens medicin [Internet]. 17 december 2019 [15/8-2022]. Available from: https://www.dagensmedicin.se/alla-nyheter/nyheter/kritiserad-larmcentral-far-vara-kvar/

29. Sjögren, Anna. Larmet inifrån SOS Alarm: Tidsfråga innan det kollapsar. Aftonbladet [Internet]. 19 decmber 2021 [15/8-2022]. Available from: https://www.aftonbladet.se/nyheter/a/Rrl9ma/larmet-inifran-sos-alarm-tidsfraga-innan-det-kollapsar

30. Fredén, Jonas. Rekordmånga larmsamtal – ett av tre i onödan. Svenska Dagbladet [Internet]. 8 augusti 2021 [15/8-2022]. Available from: https://www.svd.se/a/Eayzr3/larm-till-sos-slar-rekord

31. Karlsson, Ayla. Hjärtsjuk fick vänta på aambulans i en timme. Svt [Internet]. 10 decmeber 2017 [15 /8-2022]. Available from: https://www.svt.se/nyheter/lokalt/gavleborg/sos-far-kritik-hjartsjuk-fick-vanta-pa-ambulans-i-over-40-minuter [15 /8-2022]

32. Haupt, Inger. Patient dog i väntan på ambulans - sattes i "virtuellt väntrum". Svt [Internet]. 10 juni 2022 [15/8-2022]. Available from: https://www.svt.se/nyheter/lokalt/norrbotten/patient-forblodde-i-vantan-pa-ambulans-ringde-112-och-sattes-i-virtuellt-vantrum

33. Johansson, Otto. Bröt ryggen - blev nekad ambulans två gånger. Svt [Internet]. 17 november 2021 [15 /8-2022]. Available from: https://www.svt.se/nyheter/lokalt/skane/brot-ryggen-blev-nekad-ambulans-tva-ganger [15 /8-2022]

34. Risenfors, Kristian. Kvinna nekades ambulans flera gånger – dog. GöteborgDirekt [Internet]. 29 juni 2020 [15/8-2022]. Available from: https://www.gp.se/nyheter/g%C3%B6teborg/nekades-ambulans-tv%C3%A5-g%C3%A5nger-kvinna-dog-1.30348558

35. Doktorn. Längre väntan på ambulans idag än för fem år sedan. 2015 [28/4; 15/8 2022]. Available from: https://www.doktorn.com/artikel/l%C3%A4ngre-v%C3%A4ntetid-p%C3%A5-ambulans-i-dag-%C3%A4n-f%C3%B6r-fem-%C3%A5r-sedan/

36. Hermansson, Alice. Ambulans vägrade åka på coronalarm. Expressen [Internet]. 27 februari 2022 [15/8-2022]. Available from: https://www.expressen.se/nyheter/ambulans-vagrade-aka-pa-coronalarm/

37. Kristoffersson, Simon. Ambulans vägrade ta emot larm – patient fick vänta i flera timmar. Samnytt [Internet]. 23 februari 2020 [15/8-2022]. Available from: https://samnytt.se/ambulanspersonal-vagrade-ta-emot-larm-patient-fick-vanta-flera-timmar/

38. Roos, Jimmy. Fel informatiuon till ambulansen – nådde inte ansvarig läkare. Svt [Internet]. 26 juli 2018 [15/8-2022]. Available from: https://www.svt.se/nyheter/lokalt/gavleborg/fel-information-till-ambulansen-nadde-inte-ansvarig-lakare

39. Roos, Jimmy. Ambulans gick på lunch - svårt skadad fick vänta.. Svt [Internet]. 4 juni 2018 [15/8-2022]. https://www.svt.se/nyheter/lokalt/gavleborg/ambulanspersonal-gick-pa-lunch-svart-skadad-fick-vanta

40. Engelro, Erik. Ambulanspersonal straffas – en sparkas. Svt [Internet]. 14 mars 2018 [15/8-2022]. https://www.svt.se/nyheter/lokalt/gavleborg/ambulanspersonal-straffas-en-sparkas

41. Engelro, Erik. Ambulans missade larma akuten – patient avled. 18 september 2017 [15/8-2022]. Available from: https://www.svt.se/nyheter/lokalt/gavleborg/ambulans-missade-larma-akuten-patient-avled

42. Lünning, Sanna. Ambulanspersonal: Vi kommer inte att klara julen. Svt [Internet]. 3 januari 2022 [15/8-2022]. Available from: https://www.svt.se/nyheter/lokalt/stockholm/ambulanspersonal-vi-kommer-inte-klara-julen

43. Johansson, Emma. Längre väntan på ambulans i östra länsdelarna. Svt [Internet]. 16 juni 2022 [15/8-2022]. Available from: https://www.svt.se/nyheter/lokalt/jonkoping/langre-vantan-pa-ambulans-pa-hoglandet

44. Carpman, Annika. Längre väntan på ambulans vid hjärtstopp. Dagens medicin [Internet]. 15 juni 2021 [15/8-2022].. Available from: https://www.dagensmedicin.se/specialistomraden/hjarta-karl/langre-vantan-pa-ambulans-vid-hjartstopp/

45. Kristoffersson, Simon. William tvingades vänta flera timmar på ambulans. Samnytt [Internet]. 27 januari 2020 [15 /8-2022]. Available from: https://samnytt.se/william-tvingades-vanta-flera-timmar-pa-ambulans/

46. Lång, Elisabeth. Kördes inte till sjukhus efter fall – trots hjärnblödning. Svt [Internet]. 22 januari 2020 [15 /8-2022]. https://www.svt.se/nyheter/lokalt/norrbotten/kordes-inte-till-sjukhus-efter-fall-hade-hjarnblodning

47. Lundbäck, Annica. Mindre än hälften av de asylsökande fick hälsoundersökning 2015. Läkartidningen. 19 september 2016 [15/8-2022]. Available from: https://lakartidningen.se/aktuellt/nyheter/2016/09/mindre-an-halften-av-de-asylsokande-fick-halsoundersokning-2015/

48. Folkhälsomyndigheten. Tuberkulos – sjukdomsstatistik [Internet]. [15/8-2022]. Available from: https://www.fohm.se/folkhalsorapportering-statistik/statistik-a-o/sjukdomsstatistik/tuberkulos/?p=48740

49. Atterstam, Inger. Somalier oroas av autismlarm. Svenska dagbladet. 7 november 2009 [15/8-2022]. https://www.svd.se/a/a7b14592-3b57-3715-8a0f-831bbf749127/somalier-oroas-av-autismlarm

50. Ingvarsson, Cecilia. Falska rykten ligger bakom nytt mässlingsutbrott. Svt. 17 mars 2017 [15/8-2022]. Available from: https://www.svt.se/nyheter/lokalt/stockholm/falska-rykten-kan-ligga-bakom-nytt-masslingsutbrott

51. Liljeborg, Lena. Rekordmånga smittade av resistenta bakterier. Svt. 14 januari 2017 [18/8-2022]. Available from: https://www.svt.se/nyheter/lokalt/ost/rekordmanga-smittades-av-mrsa-och-esbl-under-2016

52. Nyhaga, Michael. Risk för MRSA-smitta problem för vårdanställda. Suntarbetsliv. 2007 [18/8-2022]. Available from: https://www.suntarbetsliv.se/artiklar/sam/risk-for-mrsa-smitta-problem-for-vardanstallda/

53. Gustafsson, Eva B; Melander, Eva; Johansson, P J Hugo. MRSA-spridning på vårdcentraler. Läkartidningen. 7 maj 2013 [18/8-2022]. Available from: https://lakartidningen.se/klinik-och-vetenskap-1/artiklar-1/rapport/2013/05/mrsa-spridning-pa-vardcentraler/

54. Region Stockholm. MRSA ökar i samhället. 2018 [18/8-2022].
Available from:
https://janusinfo.se/nyheter/tidningenevidens/nr52017temainfektioner/5/mrs
aokarisamhallet.5.710ed317161746d80521f302.html

55. Björkqvist, Kent. Resistenta bakterier ökar i Sverige. Life-time. 16 juni
2016 [18/8-2022]. Available from: https://www.life-
time.se/vardkvalitet/resistenta-bakterier-okar-i-sverige/

56. Erici, Rebecka. MRSA-fallen trefaldigade på tio år. Svt. 3 januari 2016
[18/8-2022]. Available from:
https://www.svt.se/nyheter/lokalt/skane/tredubbling-av-mrsa-fall-pa-tio-ar

57. Abraha, Billy. MRSA ökar i Västernorrland. Sveriges radio. 19 januari
2016 [18/8-2022]. Available from: https://sverigesradio.se/artikel/6346115

58. Socialdepartementet. Svensk strategi för arbete mot antibiotikaresistens.
Stockholm: Socialdepartementet. 2016 [18/8-2022]. Available from:
https://www.regeringen.se/4a8234/contentassets/7b70f26ea0e74e18ab6cd1c
c5d3f030f/svensk-strategi-for-arbetet-mot-antibiotikaresistens.pdf

59. Mirsch, Helena. Mrsa ökar i samhället – men minskar på sjukhusen.
Vårdfokus. 8 maj 2012 [18/8-2022]. Aavilable from:
https://www.vardfokus.se/patientsakerhet/mrsa-okar-i-samhallet-men-
minskar-pa-sjukhusen/

60. Forskning.se. MRSA-smitta sker ofta utomlands. 22 februari 2006 [18/8-
2022]. https://www.forskning.se/2006/02/22/mrsa-smitta-sker-ofta-
utomlands/

61. Penicilin, Ingrid Lund. Resistent bakterie ökar i Sverige. 8 januari 2016
[18/8-2022]. https://penicillin.se/nyhetsinlagg/resistent-bakterie-okar-i-
sverige/

62. Andersson, Matilda. Väntetiden upp till sex år till Folktandvården.
Sveriges Radio. 28 mars 2021 [27/8-2021]. Available from:
https://sverigesradio.se/artikel/vantetiden-upp-till-sex-ar-for-tandlakartid

63. Krey, Jens. Kirurger slår larm om resursbrist. Dagens Medicin. 3 mars
2017 [27/8-2021]. Available from:
https://www.dagensmedicin.se/specialistomraden/kirurgi/kirurger-slar-larm-
om-resursbrist/

64. Galinon, Vivien. Läkaren slår larm om cancerköerna. Expressen [Internet]. 8 februari 2022 [27/8-2021]. Aavilable from:
https://www.expressen.se/kvallsposten/lakaren-slar-larm--om-cancerkoerna/

65. Nyström, Ulf.. Svenska patienter har längst väntetid i Europa. Göteborgsposten. 3 december 2013 [27/8-2021]. Available from:
https://www.gp.se/nyheter/sverige/svenska-patienter-har-l%C3%A4ngst-v%C3%A4ntetid-i-europa-1.614097

66. Franchell, Eva. Patienterna dör i väntan på sängar. Aftonbladet [Internet]. 9 maj2017[27/8-2021]. Available from:
https://www.aftonbladet.se/ledare/a/Wpd2d/patienterna-dor-i-vantan-pa-sangar

67. Mary Mårtensson. Så länge får män med prostatacancer vänta på operation [Internet]. Wellness: 2019 [27/8-2021]. Available from:
https://www.wellness.se/underliv/prostata/a/nAL7nm/sa-lange-far-man-med-prostatacancer-vanta-pa-operation

68. Lagercrantz, Maja. Delvis sant att vårdköerna har fördubblats. Sveriges radio. 25 april 2018 [27/8-2021]. Available from:
https://sverigesradio.se/artikel/6936909

69. Nyberg, Micke. Läkare slår larm om inställda operationer: "Kan handla om liv eller död för patienterna". Svt. 10 juni 2021. Available from:
https://www.svt.se/nyheter/lokalt/norrbotten/lakare-slar-larm-om-installda-operationer-det-kan-handla-om-liv-eller-dod-for-patienterna [27/8-2021]

70. Sundén, Erica. Läkare slår larm: Hyrstopp stoppar operationer. Svt. 18 September 2018 [27/8-2021]. Available from:
https://www.svt.se/nyheter/lokalt/norrbotten/lakare-slar-larm-hyrstopp-stoppar-operationer

71. Lundbäck, Annica. 10 000 inställda operationer i Stockholm förra året. Läkartidningen. 6 november 2017 [27/8-2021]. Available from:
https://lakartidningen.se/aktuellt/nyheter/2017/11/10-000-installda-operationer-i-stockholm-forra-aret/

72. TT; Dagens Medicin. Cancerpatienter får opereras utomlands. Dagens Medicin. 21 november 2019 [27/8-2021]. Available from:
https://www.dagensmedicin.se/specialistomraden/cancer/cancerpatienter-far-opereras-utomlands/

73. Mirsch, Helena. Vårdfokus. Sjuksköterskebrist tvingade patient åka till Tyskland för akut canceroperation. 22 Augusti 2018 [27/8-2021]. Available from:
https://www.vardfokus.se/yrkesroller/sjukskoterska/sjukskoterskebrist-tvingade-patient-aka-till-tyskland-for-akut-canceroperation/

74. Andersson, Joakim. Läkartidningen. Läkare lägger en dag i veckan på administration. 3 juli 2019 [20/8-2022]. Available from:
https://lakartidningen.se/aktuellt/nyheter/2019/07/lakare-lagger-en-dag-i-veckan-pa-administration/

75. Thornblad, Helene. Sjukhusläkaren. Så ska läkare avlastas administrativ arbetsbörda. 12 april 2012 [20/8-2022]. Available from:
https://www.sjukhuslakaren.se/sa-ska-lakare-avlastas-administrativ-arbetsborda/

76. Lundgren, Hans. Du&jobbet. Därför begravs vi allt mer i pappersarbete.. 25 Maj 2016 [20/8-2022]. Available from:
https://www.duochjobbet.se/article_archive/darfor-begravs-vi-allt-mer-i-pappersarbete/

77. Mellgren, Fredrik. Svenska dagbladet. Tusentals dör av felbehandling. 30 januari 2006 [21/9-2022]. Available from:
https://www.svd.se/a/5fd784bd-f6ae-35a1-a1df-1084b37c0686/tusentals-dor-av-felbehandling

78. Kallin, Jenny. Vårdfokus. Många dör i onödan av vårdskador. 29 april. 2019 [21/9-2022]. Available from:
https://www.vardfokus.se/patientsakerhet/manga-dor-i-onodan-av-vardskador/

79. P4 Västernorrland. Sveriges radio. Patient avled på sjukhus – personer blockerade livräddningsutrustning. 29 december 2021 [21/9-2022]. Available from: https://sverigesradio.se/artikel/patient-avled-pa-sjukhus-personer-blockerade-livraddningsutrustning

80. Lundmark, Viktor; Nilsson, Ellika. Svt. Ung man dog på sjukhuset efter lång väntan på vård. 19 december 2018 [21/9-2022]. Available from:
https://www.svt.se/nyheter/lokalt/norrbotten/ung-man-dog-pa-akuten-efter-lang-vantan-pa-vard

81. Svenska Dagbladet. LO-basen: Flyktingar kan ge Sverige superekonomi. 16 december 2015 [28/8-2022]. Available from: https://www.svd.se/a/1342c9a5-e7db-49cb-bc8c-3e871b02dee3/lo-basen-flyktingar-kan-ge-sverige-superekonomi

82. Fria Tider [Internet]. Expressen-krönikör: "Nu kollapsar välfärden". 4 januari 2020 [28/8-2022]. https://www.friatider.se/expressen-kronikor-nu-kollapsar-valfarden

83. Fria Tider [Internet]. Gävle tog emot "många nyanlända" – nu rasar välfärden. 18 februari 2020 [28/8-2022]. Available from: https://www.friatider.se/gavle-tog-emot-manga-nyanlanda-nu-rasar-valfarden

84. Fria Tider. Kommunernas skulder ökar till 726 miljarder: "Befolkningen växer". 13 oktober 2020 [28/8-2022]. Available from: https://www.friatider.se/kommunernas-skulder-okar-till-726-miljarder-befolkningen-vaxer

85. Fria Tider. Asylnotan: Höjd skatt i 61 kommuner vid nyår trots kraftigt minskad välfärd. 18 december 2019 [28/8-2022]. Available from: https://www.friatider.se/skatten-h-js-i-61-kommuner-vid-ny-r

86. Ulander, Kenneth. svt. Lista: Så sparar kommunerna. 26 Januari 2020 [28/8-2022]. Available from: https://www.svt.se/nyheter/inrikes/lista-sa-sparar-kommunerna

87. Fria Tider. Efter invandringen: Välfärden i Filipstad på väg att kollapsa. 1 februari 2020 [28/8-2022]. Available from: https://www.friatider.se/efter-invandringen-valfarden-i-filipstad-pa-vag-att-kollapsa

88. Bergström, Bengt. Norran. Varför betalar kommunen körkort till ensamkommande unga flyktingar?. 12 Oktober 2016 [28/8-2022]. Available from: https://norran.se/asikter/insandare/varfor-betalar-kommunen-korkort-till-ensamkommande-unga-flyktingar-677883

89. Fria Tider. Skräcksiffrorna från Uppsala: Invandring får socialbidrag att skena. 1 oktober 2019 [28/8-2022]. Available from: https://www.friatider.se/skr-cksiffrorna-fr-n-uppsala-invandring-f-r-socialbidrag-att-skena

90. Nilsson, Helena Bohm; Nyqvist, Oskar. Svt. Var fjärde svensk kommun har vuxit av invandringen. 18 Februari 2020 [28/8-2022]. Available from: https://www.svt.se/nyheter/lokalt/skane/ostra-goinge-har-vuxit-med-utrikes-fodda

91. Maja Aase, Nätverket för Gynekologisk cancer. Svårt få ersättning för vård utomlands [Internet]. [4/9-2022]. Available from: https://gyncancer.se/2014/04/svart-fa-ersattning-for-vard-utomlands/

92. Olofsson, Johanna. Expressen [Internet]. Vården missade pojkes hjärntumör – i sex år. 9 juni 2021. [4/9-2022]. Availablr from: https://www.expressen.se/kvallsposten/varden-missade-pojkes-hjarntumor-i-sex-ars-tid/

93. Vickhoff, Alexander. Aftonbladet [Internet]. Vårdcentral missade flickans hjärntumör. 7 september 2016 [4/9-2022]. Available from: https://www.expressen.se/kvallsposten/vardcentral-missade-flickans-hjarntumor/

94. Strömberg, Lars-Olof. Expressen [Internet]. Fyraåring blev blind efter sjukhusvård. 17 januari 2020 [4/9-2022]. Available from: https://www.expressen.se/kvallsposten/fyraaring-blev-blind-efter-sjukhusvard/

95. Holm, Gusten. Expressen [Internet]. Man misstänks ha våldtagit kvinna med anorexi på Karolinska sjukhuset. 26 juni 2021 [4/9-2022]. Available from: https://www.expressen.se/nyheter/man-misstanks-ha-valdtagit-kvinna--med-anorexi-pa-karolinska-sjukhuset/

96. Klugman, Olof. Tidningensyre. Privat sjukförsäkring kan ha räddat cancersjuka Angelicas liv: "Skyldig att berätta". 18 december 2020 [4/9-2022]. Available from: https://tidningensyre.se/2020/18-december-2020/vard-pa-olika-villkor-nar-privata-forsakringar-vaxer/

97. Kuronen, Alexander. Omni. Hjärtsjuk 2-åring andas via rör – nekas assistans. 26 augusti 2018 [4/9-2022]. Available from: https://omni.se/hjartsjuk-2aring-andas-via-ror-nekas-assistans/a/a2EA72

98. TT. Svenska Dagbladet. 23 dagar efter BB stängdes – första förlossningen i bil. 24 Februari 2017 [4/9-2022]. Available from: https://www.svd.se/a/5apW1/23-dagar-efter-bb-stangdes-forsta-forlossningen-i-bil

99. Sällberg, Amanda. Expressen [Internet]. Ulf har lagt en miljon på behandlingar utomlands. 28 april 2019 [4/9-2022]. Available from: https://www.expressen.se/nyheter/ulf-har-lagt-en-miljon-pa-behandlingar-utomlands/

100. Blume, Ebba. Sjukhusläkaren [Internet]. Allt fler svenskar söker vård vid Docrates i Finland-där omstridd behandling nu även ges vid universitetssjukhus. 29 oktober 2018 [4/9-2022]. Available from: https://www.sjukhuslakaren.se/allt-fler-svenskar-soker-vard-vid-docrates-i-finland-dar-omstridd-behandling-nu-aven-ges-vid-universitetssjukhus/

101. Palm, Fanny. Svt [Internet]. Sjuksköterskan Catarina låg på akuten i 17 timmar. 22 juni 2017 [4/9-2022]. Available from: https://www.svt.se/nyheter/lokalt/helsingborg/catarina-lag-pa-akuten-i-sjutton-timmar

102. Kristoffersson, Simon. Samnytt [Internet]. Sjukhus nonchalerade 4-åring med blodcancer – skickades hem flera gånger med värktabletter. 30 november 2019 [4/9-2022]. Available from: https://samnytt.se/sjukhus-nonchalerade-4-aring-med-blodcancer-skickades-hem-flera-ganger-med-varktabletter/

103. Torvinen, Anne. Svt [Internet]. Hon åkte utomlands för att få cancervård – "Fått livet tillbaka". 18 December 2018 [4/9-2022]. Available from: https://www.svt.se/nyheter/lokalt/smaland/patienter-aker-utomlands-for-att-fa-cancervard

7.2.3 Sweden during WW2

5. Flam, Aron. Det här är en svensk tiger. Stockholm: Samizdat publishing. 2019.

7.2.4 It is all about *Folkhemmet*

104. Burke, Callum Patrick. Were the Nazis revolutionary or evolutionary? German Ostsiedlung to Nazi Lebensraum. Researchgate: Loughborough University; 2014; B019430.
file:///C:/Users/46709/Downloads/WeretheNazisrevolutionaryorevolutionary GermanOstsiedlungtoNaziLebensraum.pdf [23/9-2023]

7.3.1 How Sweden handled corona in the beginning
105. Tegnellcitat. Angående Covid-19 år 2020. U.Å [18/11-2021]

106. SVT Nyheter. WHO: Oklart om epidemin planar ut. Svt [Internet]. 12 februari 2020 [18/11-2021]. Available from: https://www.svt.se/nyheter/snabbkollen/who-oklart-om-epidemin-planar-ut

107. Emanuel Karlsten. Ettårskontroll av pandemin: Sverige var sist med åtgärder - eftersom Folkhälsomyndigheten inte tror att det hjälper. 2021 [6 april; 18/11-2021]. Available from: https://emanuelkarlsten.se/ettarskontroll-av-pandemin-sverige-var-sist-med-atgarder-eftersom-folkhalsomyndigheten-inte-tror-att-det-hjalper/

108. Vogel, Gretchen. Sweden´s Gamble. Science [Internet]. 6th October 2020 [30/12-2021]. Available from: https://www.science.org/content/article/it-s-been-so-so-surreal-critics-sweden-s-lax-pandemic-policies-face-fierce-backlash

109. Borget, Linnéa. Corona-rådet: Finns ingen anledning att stanna hemma trots resor. [28 februari 2020 14/11-2021]. Available from: https://skolvarlden.se/artiklar/corona-radet-finns-ingen-anledning-att-stanna-hemma-trots-resor

110. Rundberg, Hampus; Langert, Danielle. Svt [Internet]. Sportlovet slut – stockholmare kommer hem från riskområden. 29 februari 2020 [14/11-2021]. Available from: https://www.svt.se/nyheter/lokalt/stockholm/sportlovet-slut-stockholmare-kommer-hem-fran-riskomraden

111. Hagberg, Jan. Senioren [Internet]. Smittan på äldreboendena kom från alpresenärerna. 29 oktober 2021 [11/12-2021]. Available from: https://www.senioren.se/nyheter/smittan-pa-aldreboendena-kom-fran-alpresenarerna/

112. Aksoy, Mira. Samnytt [Internet]. Svenske Mickael kan bära på Corona-viruset – staten säger att det är fritt fram att komma hem. 26 januari 2020 [14/11-2021]. Available from: https://samnytt.se/svenske-mickael-kan-bara-pa-corona-viruset-smittskyddet-sager-att-det-ar-fritt-fram-att-komma-hem/

113. Paterlini, Marta. Nature [Internet]. "Closing borders is ridiculous": the epidemiologist behind Sweden's controversial coronavirus strategy. 21 april 2020 [14/11-2021]. Available from: https://www.nature.com/articles/d41586-020-01098-x

114. Fria Tider. Tegnell förespråkar "öppna gränser". 29 maj 2020 [26/12-2021]. Available from: https://www.friatider.se/tegnell-foresprakar-oppna-granser

115. Putilov, Egor. Samnytt [Interent]. Statsepidemiolog vilseledde om direktflyg från Kina: "Det spelar ingen roll". Samnytt. 30 januari 2020 [22/9-2022]. Available from: https://samnytt.se/statsepidemiolog-vilseledde-om-direktflyg-fran-kina-det-spelar-ingen-roll/

116. Radakovits, Eva; Andersson, Ida Leveby. MittiStockholm [Internet]. Inga generella coronakontroller på Arlanda. 29 februari 2020 [22/9-2022]. Available from: https://www.mitti.se/nyheter/inga-generella-coronakontroller-pa-arlanda/lmtbC!8083751/

117. Ekeroth, Kent. 2020. Fortfarande inga hälsokontroller på svenska flygplatser när utrikesflygen landar. *Samnytt*. 28 mars. https://samnytt.se/fortfarande-inga-halsokontroller-pa-svenska-flygplatser-nar-utrikesflygen-landar/ [22/9-2022]

118. Axelsson, Sofie. MittIStockholm [Online]. Därför görs inte kontroller på flygplatserna. 18 februari 2020 [22/9-2022]. Available from: https://www.mitti.se/nyheter/darfor-gors-inte-kontroller-pa-flygplatserna/reptbr!cTAvJuY3tOB8Er2PhXXIw/

119. Öhrn, Linda. Dagens industri. Folkhälsomyndigheten: Oron får företag att blunda för fakta. 5 mars 2020 [17/12-2021]. Available from: https://www.di.se/nyheter/folkhalsomyndigheten-oron-far-foretag-att-blunda-for-fakta/

120. TT / VID. VärldenIdag [Internet]. Anders Tegnell: Ingen såg det extrema komma. Världenidag. 18 januari 2021 [22/9-2022]. Available from: https://www.varldenidag.se/nyheter/anders-tegnell-ingen-sag-det-extrema-komma/reptlp!NSYQ71gMVHpSD54L4hMu8w/

121. Nordström, Isabelle. Omni [Internet]. Tegnell medger miss i virus-bedömning: "Trodde att Kina skulle få stopp på det". 7 mars 2020 [29/9-2022]. Available from: https://omni.se/tegnell-medger-miss-i-virusbedomning-trodde-att-kina-skulle-fa-stopp-pa-det/a/pLkM9E

122. TT. Aftonbladet [Internet]. Corona kan slå ut vanliga influensan. 3 februari 2020 [20/11-2021]. Available from: https://www.aftonbladet.se/nyheter/a/jd72Mb/corona-kan-sla-ut-vanliga-influensan

123. Higgins-Dunn, Noah; Lovelace Jr.,Berkeley. Top US health official says the coronavirus is 10 times 'more lethal' than the seasonal flu. CNBC [Internet]. 11 march 2020 [20/9-2022]. Available feom: https://www.cnbc.com/2020/03/11/top-federal-health-official-says-coronavirus-outbreak-is-going-to-get-worse-in-the-us.html

124. Jakobson, Hanna; Holmström, Mikael. Dagens Nyheter [Internet]. Ökningen av antalet importfall kan ha nått toppen – kommer snart att klinga av". 6 mars 2020 [20/11-2021]. Availble from: https://www.dn.se/nyheter/sverige/antalet-coronafall-i-sverige-kan-ha-natt-toppen-kommer-snart-att-klinga-av/

125. Ekroth, Benjamin. Aftonbladet [Internet]. Statsepidemiologen: Toppen kan vara nådd nu. 7 mars 2020 [20/11-2021]. Available from: https://www.aftonbladet.se/nyheter/a/RRpj0A/statsepidemiologen-toppen-kan-vara-nadd-nu

126. Yousuf, Etezaz. Göteborgsposten [Internet]. Tegnell: Dödstalen i Sverige kunde undvikits. 24 juni 2020 [29/9-2022]; Available fom: https://www.gp.se/nyheter/g%C3%B6teborg/tegnell-d%C3%B6dstalen-i-sverige-kunde-undvikits-1.30138301

127. Lewis, Evan. Newsbrig [Internet]. Swedish health expert blames COVID-19 deaths on mild flu season.. 23rd of September 2020 [30/12-2021]. Available from: https://newsbrig.com/swedish-health-expert-blames-covid-19-deaths-on-mild-flu-season/126441/

7.3.2 How Sweden recieved a natural herd immunity strategi

128. TT. NyTeknik. FHM:s tidiga strategi var flockimmunitet. 6 November 2020 [18/10-2022]. Available from: https://www.nyteknik.se/samhalle/fhm-s-tidiga-strategi-var-flockimmunitet-7004491

129. Tronarp, Gustaf. WHO: Inga bevis för att människor som haft covid-19 är immuna. Aftonbladet [Internet]. 19 april 2020 [8/9-2024]; Available from: https://www.aftonbladet.se/nyheter/a/Vb8Jj1/who-inga-bevis-for-att-manniskor-som-haft-covid-19-ar-immuna

130. Kvartoft, Camilla; Nike Nylander. Coronautfrågningen [Tv program]. Del 1. Svt: Svt; 17 januari 2021.

131. Ekblom. Jonas. Tegnell: Flockimmunitet inte huvudtaktiken. Svenska Dagbladet [Internet]. 15 mars 2020 [8/9-2024]; Available from: https://www.svd.se/a/GGmJ7l/tegnell-flockimmunitet-inte-huvudtaktiken

132. Emanuel Karlsten. Tegnell-mejlen: Berättelsen om Johan Giesecke och Folkhälsomyndigheten [Internet]. 2020 [11 august; 18/11-2021]. Available from: https://emanuelkarlsten.se/tegnell-mejlen-berattelsen-om-johan-giesecke-och-folkhalsomyndigheten/

133. Emanuel Karlsten. Tegnell-mejlen: Så fick flockimmuniteten fäste hos Folkhälsomyndigheten. 2020 [12/8; 6/1-2022]. Available from: https://emanuelkarlsten.se/tegnell-mejlen-sa-fick-flockimmuniteten-faste-hos-folkhalsomyndigheten/

134. Larsson, Petter J. Aftonbladet [Internet]. Anders Tegnell hyllar brittisk tanke kring flockimmunitet: "Dit vi behöver komma". 17 mars 2020 [18/11-2021]. Available from: https://www.aftonbladet.se/nyheter/a/6j7vaO/anders-tegnell-hyllar-brittisk-tanke-kring-flockimmunitet-dit-vi-beh

135. Frans, Emma. Svenska Dagbladet. Alla måste hjälpas åt att undvika smittan – särskilt äldre. 18 mars 2020 [18/11-2021]. Available from: https://www.svd.se/alla-maste-hjalpas-at-att-undvika-smittan--sarskilt-aldre

136. Carlsson, Tucker. Swedish ambassador to the US on her country's path to 'herd immunity' against the coronavirus. [Tv program]. New York: Fox News; 6th May. Available from: https://www.foxnews.com/transcript/swedish-ambassador-to-the-us-on-her-countrys-path-to-herd-immunity-against-the-coronavirus

137. Björkman, Karl. Nya Tider. Anders Tegnell raderade flertal mejl – kan vara lagbrott. 15 augusti 2020 [2/10-2022]. Available from: https://www.nyatider.nu/anders-tegnell-raderade-flertal-mejl-kan-vara-lagbrott/

138. Headtopics. Tegnell raderade coronamejl: "Vi slänger massa arbetsmaterial". 14 augusti 2020 [2/10-2022]. Available from: https://headtopics.com/se/tegnell-raderade-coronamejl-vi-slanger-massa-arbetsmaterial-14978886

139. Wikström, Olivia. Omni. Tegnell raderade mejl från myndigheter och experter. 14 augusti 2020 [2/10-2022]. https://omni.se/tegnell-raderade-mejl-fran-myndigheter-och-experter/a/kJAqAB

153

140. Sandberg, Mattias. Aftonbladet [Internet]. Tegnell raderade mejl från myndigheter och experter. 14 Augusti 2020 [2/10-2022]. Available from: https://www.aftonbladet.se/nyheter/a/vQ4EQ4/tegnell-raderade-mejl-fran-myndigheter-och-experter

141. Kerpner, Joachim. Aftonbladet [Internet]. Tegnell backar: "Coronakulmen på måndag eller tisdag". 8 Mars 2020 [10/10-2022]. Available from: https://www.aftonbladet.se/nyheter/a/9vdbWd/tegnell-backar-coronakulmen-pa-mandag-eller-tisdag

142. Falkirk, John. Svenska Dagbladet. Tegnell: Min bedömning om Kina visade sig inte vara rätt. 9 mars 2020 [10/10-2022]. Available from: https://www.svd.se/a/MRbAlK/min-bedomning-om-kina-visade-sig-inte-vara-ratt

143. Mossige-Norheim, Thea. Expressen [Internet]. Flera nya smittade – 180 fall Sverige. 8 mars 2020 [17/9-2024]. Available from: https://www.expressen.se/nyheter/minst-3-000-testade-for-corona-i-sverige/

144. Davies, Guy; Roeber, Bruno. abcNEWS. Sweden stayed open during the coronavirus pandemic: Is it a model for the future?. 27th May 2020 [10/10-2022]. Available from: https://abcnews.go.com/International/sweden-stayed-open-coronavirus-pandemic-model-future/story?id=70666450

145. Magnå, Joakim; Karlsson, Josefina. Tegnell: Sverige klarar hösten bättre än Norge. Expressen [Internet]. 21 juli 2020 [8/9-2024]; Available from; https://www.expressen.se/nyheter/presstraff-med-det-senaste-om-coronutbrottet/

146. Majlard, Jan. Svenska Dagbladet. Ny kalkyl: Stockholm kan nå flockimmunitet i juni 10 maj 2020 [25/12-2021]. Available from: https://www.svd.se/ny-berakning-stockholm-kan-na-immunitet-i-juni

147. Wikén, Erik. Svt. Tom Britton: Därför hade jag fel om flockimmuniteten. 3 December 2020 [25/12-2021]. Available from: https://www.svt.se/nyheter/inrikes/tom-britton-darfor-hade-jag-fel-om-flockimmuniteten

148. Ronge, Johan. Expressen [Internet]. Spridningen av coronaviruset. Efter feltrampen: Brittons nya prognos om immunitet. 28 november 2020 [25/12-2021]. Available from: https://www.expressen.se/nyheter/efter-feltrampen-brittons-nya-prognos-om-immunitet/

149. Stockholm universitet. Naturvetenskapliga fakulteten. Tom Britton får pris som Årets Statistikfrämjare 2020. 2021 [25/12-2021].
https://www.science.su.se/om-oss/nyheter/tom-britton-f%C3%A5r-pris-som-%C3%A5rets-statistikfr%C3%A4mjare-2020-1.548606

7.3.3 Why Herd immunity would not be a viable strategy

150. De Vrieze, Jop. Science. More people are getting COVID-19 twice, suggesting immunity wanes quickly in some. 18th November 2020 [25/9-2022]. Available from: https://www.science.org/content/article/more-people-are-getting-covid-19-twice-suggesting-immunity-wanes-quickly-some

151. Ellyatt, Holly. CNBC. Woman catches Covid twice within 20 days, marking a new record. 21st April 2022 [25/9-2022]. Available from: https://www.cnbc.com/2022/04/21/woman-caught-covid-twice-in-20-days-marking-a-new-record.html

152. Larsson, Petter J. Aftonbladet [Internet]. Anders Tegnell hyllar brittisk tanke kring flockimmunitet: "Dit vi behöver komma". 17 mars 2020 [18/11-2021]. Available from: https://www.aftonbladet.se/nyheter/a/6j7vaO/anders-tegnell-hyllar-brittisk-tanke-kring-flockimmunitet-dit-vi-beh

153. Öhman, Daniel; Ridderstedt, Maria. Sveriges Radio. Positiv bild kan ha bidragit till ökad smittspridning under hösten.. 13 april 2021 [10/1-2022]. Available from: https://sverigesradio.se/artikel/positiv-bild-kan-ha-bidragit-till-okad-smittspridning-under-hosten

154. Neuding, Paulina. DagensSamhälle. Vinklad regeringskampanj för Sverigebilden. 6 mars 2017 [1/1-2022]. Available from: https://www.dagenssamhalle.se/opinion/gastkronika/vinklad-regeringskampanj-for-sverigebilden/

155. Fria Tider. Ny myndighet ska rädda "Sverigebilden". 26 maj 2020 [1/1-2022]. Available from: https://www.friatider.se/ny-myndighet-ska-radda-sverigebilden

156. Torstensson, Simon. Ekonomifakta. Arbetslöshet – internationellt. 2022 [1/9; 30/9-2022]. Available from: https://www.ekonomifakta.se/fakta/arbetsmarknad/arbetsloshet/arbetsloshet--internationell-jamforelse/

157. Fria Tider [Internet]. Regeringens desperata drag: Ambassadörer pressas att rädda Sverigebilden. 3 juni 2020 [1/1-2022]. Available from: https://www.friatider.se/regeringens-desperata-drag-ambassadorer-pressas-att-radda-sverigebilden

158. Lindberg, Staffan. Aftonbladet [Internet]. Dokument avslöjar: Så försöker regeringen rädda Sverigebilden. 3 juni 2020 [7/1-2022]. Available from: https://www.aftonbladet.se/nyheter/a/kJ75LQ/dokument-avslojar-sa-forsoker-regeringen-radda-sverigebilden

159. Rootzén, Holger. Expressen [Internet]. FHM försöker dölja sitt misslyckande. 6 juli 2020 [1/1-2022]. Available from: https://www.expressen.se/debatt/fhm-forsoker-dolja-sitt-misslyckande/

160. Holmgren, Mia. Dagens nyheter [Internet]. Tegnell: Vi får oroande rapporter om trängsel i utelivet. 21 april 2020 [1/1-2022]. Available from: https://www.dn.se/nyheter/sverige/tegnell-vi-far-oroande-rapporter-om-trangsel-i-utelivet/

161. Nikel, David. Forbes. Sweden Health Agency Withdraws Controversial Coronavirus Report.. 22nd April 2020 [7/1-2022]. Available from: https://www.forbes.com/sites/davidnikel/2020/04/22/sweden-health-agency-withdraws-controversial-coronavirus-report/?sh=4a78c7484349

162. Gale, Earle. China Daily Global. Sweden says 'herd immunity' very close. 21th May 2020 [6/1-2022]. Available from: https://global.chinadaily.com.cn/a/202004/21/WS5e9e546aa3105d50a3d17a41.html

163. Larsson, Ylva. svt. Utrikesministern försvarar svenska strategin: En myt att livet pågår som vanligt. 17 April 2020 [7/1-2022]. Available from: https://www.svt.se/nyheter/inrikes/utrikesministern-forsvarar-svenska-strategin-en-myt-att-livet-pagar-som-vanligt

164. Larger, Thibault. Politico. Sweden didn't seek herd immunity to the coronavirus, top diplomat says. 4th October 2020 [7/1-2022]. Available from: https://www.politico.eu/article/sweden-coronavirus-didnt-seek-herd-immunity-torbjorn-sohlstrom/

165. Philipson, Lena. Sydsvenskan. Sju saker om corona som riskprofessorn tycker du bör känna till. 6 mars 2020 [22/9-2022]. Available from: https://www.sydsvenskan.se/2020-03-06/sju-saker-om-corona-som-riskprofessorn-tycker-du-bor-kanna-till

166. Naureckas, Jim. Fair. By 'as Successful as Most Other Nations,' NYT Means Sweden Is 10th Worst in the World. 30th April 2020 [22/9-2022]. Available from: https://fair.org/home/by-as-successful-as-most-other-nations-nyt-means-sweden-is-10th-worst-in-the-world/

167. TT; VID. Världenidag. Anders Tegnell: Ingen såg det extrema komma. 18 januari 2021 [22/9-2022]. Available from: https://www.varldenidag.se/nyheter/anders-tegnell-ingen-sag-det-extrema-komma/reptlp!NSYQ71gMVHpSD54L4hMu8w/

7.4.2 Censoration

168. Putilov, Egor. Samnytt. AVSLÖJAR: Här anmäler
Folkhälsomyndigheten coronakritiker till MSB – som agenter åt främmande
makt. 10 maj 2021 [27/8-2021]. Available from: https://samnytt.se/avslojar-
har-anmaler-folkhalsomyndigheten-coronakritiker-till-msb-som-agenter-at-
frammande-makt/

169. Hegarty, Stephanie. BBC. The Chinese doctor who tried to warn others
about coronavirus. 6th February [26/9-2022]. Available from:
https://www.bbc.com/news/world-asia-china-51364382

170. Pettersson, Mikael Grill. Svt. Kritiserade myndigheten om sågade
munskydds-utspelet: "Kunde ha varit bättre att avstå". 3 oktober 2020 [5/12-
2021]. Available from: https://www.svt.se/nyheter/inrikes/sjalvkritik-om-
sagade-munskydds-utspelet-om-munskydden-kunde-ha-varit-battre-att-avsta

171. Pettersson, Mikael Grill. Svt. Myndigheten ville slippa "svår debatt"
om munskydden – framgår av raderat mejl. 30 maj 2020 [5/12-2021].
Available from: https://www.svt.se/nyheter/inrikes/kritiserade-myndigheten-
ville-slippa-svar-debatt-om-munskydden-framgar-av-mejl-som-raderats

172. Malm, Victor. Expressen [Internet]. Coronahaveristerna är en skam för
Sverige. 15 april 2020 [5/12-2021]. Available from:
https://www.expressen.se/kultur/victor-malm/coronahaveristerna-ar-en-
skam-for-sverige/

173. Veum, Eirik. Nrk. Sverige: Koronakritikere blir spyttet på. 15 juni.
2020 [5/12-2021]. Available from: https://www.nrk.no/urix/sverige_-
koronakritikere-blir-spyttet-pa-1.15052904

174. Eriksson, Isabelle. NB Nyhetsbyrån. Sjuksköterska fick sparken efter
larm om att äldre nekas syrgas. 5 maj 2020 [01/01-2022]. Available from:
https://nyhetsbyran.org/2020/05/05/sjukskoterska-fick-sparken-efter-larm-
om-att-aldre-nekas-syrgas/

175. Samnytt. Kommun vägrade berätta om smittuppgifter: "Skulle öka oron
hos invånarna". 19 juni 2020 [01/01-2021]. Available from:
https://d5fe351e3d.nxcli.net/kommun-vagrade-beratta-om-smittuppgifter-
skulle-oka-oron-hos-invanarna/

176. Wong, Ola. Kvartal. FHM drar hatkortet. 14 Mars 2021 [10/1-2022].
Available from: https://kvartal.se/artiklar/fhm-drar-hatkortet/

177. Granström, Klas. Journalisten. Kritisk granskning av strategin dröjde – redaktioner ångrar sig. 11 Mars 2021 [10/1-2022]. Available from: https://www. journalisten.se/nyheter/kritisk-granskning-av-strategin-drojde-redaktioner-angrar-sig

178. Dahlgren, Peter. Backend Media. SVT Rapports Y-axel som inte slutade växa (covid-19). 21 februari 2021 [10/1-2022]. Available from: https://www.backendmedia.se/2021/02/21/svt-diagram/

179. Burman, Eva. Ekuriren. Eva Burman: Varför fortsätta mörka när trovärdigheten står på spel. 16 januari 2021 [6/9-2022]. Available from: https://ekuriren.se/kronika/artikel/varfor-fortsatta-morka-nar-trovardigheten-star-pa-spel/jpkgxd7r

180. Fria Tider. Politiker ljög om att Karolinska gav alla coronasjuka vård. 22 juni 2020 [6/9-2022]. Available from: https://www.friatider.se/politiker-ljog-om-att-karolinska-gav-alla-coronasjuka-vard

181. Söderberg-Nauclér, Cecilia; Brusselaers, Nele; Helander, Per; Olsen, Björn; Svensson, Jakob. Svenska Dagbladet. "Bortse inte från de bästa forskarnas modeller". 13 april 2020 [27/9-2022]. Available from: https://www.svd.se/a/0nyqA2/bortse-inte-fran-de-basta-forskarnas-modeller

182. Svensson, Olof. Professor vill se nedstängning av Stockholm. Aftonbladet [Internet]. 15 april 2020 [27/9-2022]. Available from: https://www.aftonbladet.se/nyheter/a/4qeKx6/professor-vill-se-nedstangning-av-stockholm

183. Emanuell Karlsen. Forskare förnekar önskan om Tegnells avgång – motbevisas av inspelning. 2020 [15/4; 27/9-2022]. Available from: https://emanuelkarlsten.se/forskare-fornekar-krav-om-tegnells-avgang-motbevisas-av-inspelning

184. Örstadius, Kristoffer; Ewald, Hugo. Dagens Nyheter [Internet]. Socialstyrelsen hemlighåller vårdens kapacitet att hantera ett coronavirusutbrott. 28 februari 2020 [28/9-2022]. Available from: https://www.dn.se/nyheter/sverige/socialstyrelsen-hemlighaller-vardens-kapacitet-att-hantera-ett-coronavirusutbrott/

7.4.3 The elderly

185. Pensionsmyndigheten. 2020. *Anslagbelastning och prognoser för Pensionsmyndighetens anslag*. Available from;
file:///C:/Users/46709/Downloads/Anslagsbelastning%20och%20prognoser%20f%C3%B6r%20Pensionsmyndighetens%20anslag.%20Budget%C3%A5ren%202020-2023.pdf [10/9-2022]

186. Begg, Keith; Flyg, Virpi. 2022. How Swedish authorities worked to export "herd immunity" to other countries. *Worldsocialistwebsite*. 5 June.
https://www.wsws.org/en/articles/2022/06/06/swed-j06.html [15/10-2022]

187. Kvartoft, Camilla; Nike Nylander. Coronautfrågningen [Tv program]. Del 2. Svt: Svt; 17 januari 2021.

188. Svedala kommun. (2020). Covid-team inom hemtjänsten.
https://www.svedala.se/paverka/nyheter/2020/maj/covid-team-inom-hemtjansten/ [25/8-2021]

189. Rosén, Peter A. 2021. Larm från äldreomsorgspersonal i Oskarshamns kommun: "Gör ont i hjärtat". *Oskarshamn-nytt*. 18 Oktober.
https://www.oskarshamns-nytt.se/larm-fran-aldreomsorgspersonal-i-oskarshamns-kommun-gor-ont-i-hjartat/ [9/11-2021]

190. Ohlin, Elisabet. 2020. Geriatrikprofessor: Många äldre dör i onödan utan korrekt bedömning. *Läkartidningen*. 18 maj.
https://lakartidningen.se/aktuellt/nyheter/2020/05/geriatrikprofessor-manga-aldre-dor-i-onodan-utan-korrekt-bedomning/ [27/8-2021]

191. Tångeberg, Johannes; Sundberg, Roger. 2020. 90 procent vårdas inte på sjukhus – dör på äldreboendet. *Kkuriren*. 20 maj. https://kkuriren.se/sa-manga-ar-smittade-inom-aldreomsorgen-just-nu/7r3n00ej/artikel/90-procent-vardas-inte-pa-sjukhus--dor-pa-aldreboendet/4lq2m88l [11/12-2021]

192. Österstam, Joacim. 2017. 40 000 undernärda inom äldreomsorgen. *Svenska dagbladet*. 17 april. https://www.svd.se/a/QvQGR/40-000-undernarda-inom-aldreomsorgen [30/9-2022]

193. Fallenius, Karin. 2020. Nekades intensivvård trots ledig plats – deras pappa dog i covid-19 *svt*. 12 juni.
https://www.svt.se/nyheter/lokalt/sodertalje/broderna-forlorade-sin-pappa-i-covid-19-fick-inte-intensivvard [27/8-2021]

194. Schau, Oscar; Wikén, Johan; Ulander, Kenneth. 2020. IVO: Allvarliga brister inom äldrevården under pandemin. *Svt*. 25 November. https://www.svt.se/nyheter/inrikes/ivo-allvarliga-brister-i-aldrevarden-under-pandemin [10/1-2022]

7.4.4 Systemic complications
195. Sveriges kommuner och regioner. Vanliga frågor om utjämningssystemet. 2021 [16/3;17/8-2021]Available froom: https://skr.se/skr/ekonomijuridik/ekonomi/utjamningssystem/vanligafragoro mutjamningssystemet.11892.html

196. Dorian, Hampus. Göteborgsposten. Kommunanställda vägras hemarbete: "Utsätts för smittorisk". 5 april 2020 [10/1-2022]. Available from: https://www.gp.se/nyheter/g%C3%B6teborg/kommunanst%C3%A4llda-v%C3%A4gras-hemarbete-uts%C3%A4tts-f%C3%B6r-smittorisk-1.26363810

197. Hannu, Filip. Svt. Smittskyddsläkaren i Norrbotten fick nej av Folkhälsomyndigheten. 28 maj 2021 [6/1-2022]. Available from: https://www.svt.se/nyheter/lokalt/norrbotten/nystedt-ville-ha-lokala-restriktioner-folkhalsomyndigheten-sa-nej

7.4.5 Government crisis
198. Knutsson, Mats. Svt. MP pressas i migrationsfrågan – kan lämna regeringen. 28 juni 2020 [15/8-2021]. Available from: https://www.svt.se/nyheter/inrikes/mp-pressas-i-migrationsfragan-kan-lamna-regeringen

199. Knutsson, Mats. Svt. Analys: MP:s besked kan bädda för regeringskris. 5 september 2020 [14/8-2021]. Available from: https://www.svt.se/nyheter/inrikes/mp-s-besked-kan-badda-for-regeringskris

200. Kristerson, Ulf. Aftonbladet [Internet]. Löfven har lagt sig platt för Miljöpartiet. 12 oktober 2020 [15/8-2021]. Available from: https://www.aftonbladet.se/debatt/a/R9Rj3W/lofven-har-lagt-sig-platt-for-miljopartiet

201. Knutsson, Mats. Svt [Internet]. Analys: Nya MP-statsråden kastas direkt in i hetluften. 5 februari 2020 [15/8-2021].

https://www.svt.se/nyheter/inrikes/nya-mp-statsraden-kastas-direkt-in-i-hetluften

202. Falkirk, John & Lundqvist, Axel. Expressen [Internet]. S öppnar för att ändra migrationsförslaget. 7 feb 2021 [15/8-2021]. Available from: https://www.expressen.se/nyheter/s-oppnar-for-att-andra-migrationsforslaget/

203. Expressen [Internet]. S har kapitulerat för MP om migrationen. 7 oktober 2020 [15/8-2021]. Available from: https://www.expressen.se/ledare/s-har-kapitulerat-for-mp-om-migrationen/

204. Knutsson, Mats. Svt [Internet]. Las-frågan kan snabbt eskalera till en regeringskris. 30 september 2020 [4/8-2020]. Available from: https://www.svt.se/nyheter/inrikes/las-fragan-kan-snabbt-eskalera-till-en-regeringskris

205. Klepke, Martin. 2020. Martin Klepke: Strävar arbetsgivarna efter en regeringskris i las-förhandlingarna?. *ARBETET*. 25 september. https://arbetet.se/2020/09/25/stravar-arbetsgivaren-efter-en-regeringskris-i-las-forhandlingarna/ [4/8-2020]

206. Riks. Sverigedemokraterna har väckt misstroendeförklaring mot Stefan Löfven. [Video fil]. 2021, 17 juni [23/7-2021]. Available from: https://www.youtube.com/watch?v=gR5l1FXdS2Y

207. Bostadslistan. Vad är marknadshyra och är det positivt eller negativt?. [30/9-2022]. Available from: https://bostadslistan.se/blog/marknadshyra

208. Andersson, Marja. Svt. Vad är en misstroendeförklaring?. 23 juni 2021 [11/9-2022]. Available from: https://www.svt.se/nyheter/nyhetstecken/vad-ar-en-misstroendeforklaring-1

209. Riks. Nu finns det en riksdagsmajoritet för att fälla Stefan Löfven. [Video fil]. 2021, 17 juni [23/7-2021]. Available from https://www.youtube.com/watch?v=gfnqY8pZTWU

210. Riks. En riksdagsmajoritet vill nu fälla Stefan Löfvens regering [Video fil]. 2021, 17 juni [25/7-2021]. Available from: https://www.youtube.com/watch?v=kGXwFsN1CdA

211. Riks. Efter Stefan Löfvens fall: Nu sitter kontroversiella Peter Hultqvist löst. [Video fil]. 2021, 21 juni [25/7-2021]. Available from: https://www.youtube.com/watch?v=dyuyYgBrPok

212. Aftonbladet [Internet]. Statsminister Stefan Löfven fälld av riksdagen – detta händer nu [Video fil]. 2021, 21 juni [25/7-2021]. Availeble from: https://www.youtube.com/watch?v=g_j88RHg7Ek

213. Riks. Chang Frick: Stefan Löfven försöker köpa sig tid. [Video fil]. 2021, 21 juni [29/7-2021]. Available from: https://www.youtube.com/watch?v=183q9wwTUwA

214. Aftonbladet. C backar från hyresförslag – vill ha nya förhandlingar om januariavtalet [Video fil]. 2021, 24 juni [29/7-2021]. Available from: https://www.dn.se/sverige/c-backar-fran-hyresforslag-vill-ha-nya-forhandlingar-om-januariavtalet/

215. Riks. Kommer Stefan Löfven tillbaka? Vad händer med regeringskrisen? [Video fil]. 24 juni, 2021 [25/7-2021]. Available from: https://www.youtube.com/watch?v=yxp-H6MX5nU

216. Riks. Stefan Löfven avgår - Riks förklarar vad som händer nu. [Video fil]. 28 juni, 2021 [25/7-2021]. Available from: https://www.youtube.com/watch?v=cl5NnUm0bqs

217. Riks. Löfven planerar avgång om budgeten faller. [Video fil]. 29 juni, 2021 [25/7-2021]. Available from: https://www.youtube.com/watch?v=_igfULUZ8-4

218. Riks. Intervju med Henrik Vinge, om misstroendeförklaringen mot Stefan Löfven. [Video fil]. 2021, 17 juni [23/7-2021]. Available from: https://www.youtube.com/watch?v=PFW13_VoZhc

219. Riks. Idag röstar riksdagen om Stefan Löfven. [Video fil]. 7 juli, 2021 [25/7-2021].
Available from: https://www.youtube.com/watch?v=Uht0fjAaF5k

220. Riks. Mattias Karlsson: S försökte få en statsminister genom stöd till kurdiskt kommunistparti. 2021, 24 november [20/12-2021]. https://www.youtube.com/watch?v=eyLV7k87pyM

221. Riks. Kommer Miljöpartiet hoppa av regeringen? Sverige styrs av en SD-budget. 24 novmeber, 2021 [20/12-2021]. Available from: https://www.youtube.com/watch?v=ru6PCif8JR8&_JAFnYmM6gQ5LP

222. Riks. Snälla Miljöpartiet, lämna regeringen och sedan lämna riksdagen för gott. 24 novmeber, 2021 [20/12-2021]. Available from: https://www.youtube.com/watch?v=M0IVJBlGziw

223. Riks. Socialdemokraterna har lurat Annie Lööf. [Video fil]. 24 november, 2021 [20/12-2021]. https://www.youtube.com/watch?v=DLJHrE-jTpQ

224. Riks. Miljöpartiet hoppar av regeringen - På grund av SD:s budgetvinst. [Video fil]. 24 november, 2021 [20/12-2021]. Available from: https://www.youtube.com/watch?v=GmtFBJO57qY

225. Riks. Annie Lööf blev lurad och Magdalena Andersson fick avgå. [Video fil]. 25 november, 2021 [20/12-2021]. Available from: https://www.youtube.com/watch?v=3ZZOqTcy8G0

226. Riks. Magdalena Andersson (S) vald till statsminister – igen [Video fil]. 29 november, 2021 [20/12-2021]. Available from: https://www.youtube.com/watch?v=6_4Sere2OTk

7.4.6 Covid-19 Statistics

227. Adamaltmejd. Confirmed daily Covid-19 deats in Sweden [Internet]. 2022 [26/9-2022]. Available from: http://adamaltmejd.se/covid/

228. Iselidh, Astrid; TT. Region Uppsalas covidsiffror kan ge missvisande bild. Svt. 14 januari 2022 [26/9-2024]. Available from: https://www.svt.se/nyheter/lokalt/uppsala/region-uppsalas-covidstatistik-kan-ge-missvisande-bild

229. Mathieu, Edouard. Why do COVID-19 deaths in Sweden's official data always appear to decrease?. Ourworldindata. 13th November 2020 [26/9-2022]. Available from: https://ourworldindata.org/covid-sweden-death-reporting

230. Hagberg, Sebastian. Stor eftersläpning i de svenska officiella dödstalen. Omni. 5 april 2020 [26/9-2022]. Available from: https://omni.se/stor-efterslapning-i-de-svenska-officiella-dodstalen/a/RRemWx

7.5. Corona

231. Svärd, Fanny. Tegnell: "Man måste tänka efter väldigt ordentligt". Svt [Internet]. 7 mars 2021 [8/9-2024]; Available from; https://www.svt.se/nyheter/inrikes/tegnell-4

232. Lundqvist, Axel. Annie Lööfs krav: Stäng ner samhället 2-3 veckor. Expressen [Internet]. 7 mars 2021 [8/9-2024]; Available from; https://www.expressen.se/nyheter/annie-loofs-krav-stang-ner-samhallet-2-3-veckor/

7.5.2 Tegnell on facial masks

233. Edwards, Catherine. 2020. Why is Sweden still not asking people to wear face masks?. *The Local*. 8th June.
https://www.thelocal.se/20200608/why-isnt-sweden-asking-people-to-wear-face-masks/ [1/1-2022]

234. Rönnqvist, Linnea; Sandén, Tilda. 2020. Direktören om att jobba utan munskydd: "Förstår personalens oro". *Göteborgsposten*. 26 mars.
https://www.gp.se/nyheter/g%C3%B6teborg/direkt%C3%B6ren-om-att-jobba-utan-munskydd-f%C3%B6rst%C3%A5r-personalens-oro-1.25978475 [16/2-2021]

235. Franssen, Anne Grietje. 2020. Why is Sweden not recommending face masks to the public?. *The local*. 14th May.
https://www.thelocal.se/20200514/explained-why-is-sweden-not-recommending-face-masks-to-the-public/ [16/12-2021]

236. Emanuel Karlsten. 2020. *Arbetsmiljöverket stoppar svenskar som vill hjälpa sjukvården med skyddsvisir: "Känns helt sjukt"*.
https://emanuelkarlsten.se/hundratals-svenskar-gor-3d-printade-skyddsvisir-till-sjukvarden-forbjuds-av-arbetsmiljoverket/ [17/12-2021]

237. Emanuel Karlsten. 2020. *Efter Arbetsmiljöverkets stopp för skyddsvisir – Region Skåne hittar kryphål: "Andra regioner får gärna kopiera oss"*.
https://emanuelkarlsten.se/efter-arbetsmiljoverkets-stopp-region-skane-hittar-kryphal-andra-regioner-far-garna-kopiera-oss/ [17/12-2021]

238. Fria Tider [Internet]. 2020. Attendo krossade corona med munskydd – men FHM vägrar ändra sig. 4 juli. https://www.friatider.se/attendo-krossade-corona-med-munskydd-men-fhm-vagrar-andra-sig [24/9-2022]

7.5.3 Denying herd immunity strategy

239. Ulfvarson, Daniel. Kontroversiell strategi kan minska spridningen. Svt. 15 Mars 2020 [6/1-2022]. Available from: https://www.svt.se/nyheter/inrikes/kontroversiell-strategi-kan-minska-spridningen

240. Al Jazeera. Sweden ambassador: Stockholm could reach herd immunity by May. 27th April 2020 [6/1-2022]. Available from: https://www.aljazeera.com/news/2020/4/27/sweden-ambassador-stockholm-could-reach-herd-immunity-by-may

7.5.4 Schools

241. Wigen, Malin. Föräldrar och förskollärare i bråk om coronaråden. Aftonbladet [Internet]. 4 november 2020 [7/1-2022]. Available from: https://www.aftonbladet.se/family/a/vAAblm/foraldrar-och-forskollarare-i-brak-om-coronaraden

242. Nord, Annette; Nörthen, Katrin; Jansson, Anki; Järking, Annica; Lindström, Moncia; Hall, Diana. Expressen [Internet]. Vissa föräldrar tar noll ansvar mot coronaspridningen. 31 mars 2020 [7/1-2022]. Available from: https://www.expressen.se/debatt/vissa-foraldrar-tar-noll-ansvar-mot-coronaspridningen-/

243. Gunnarsson, Helena. Arbetet. Så svarar Folkhälsomyndigheten om covid-19 i förskolan. 10 December 2020 [7/1-2022]. Available from: https://ka.se/2020/12/10/sa-svarar-folkhalsomyndigheten-om-covid-19-i-forskolan/

244. Sveriges radio [Internet]. Föräldrar som håller barn hemma i coronatider kan få böter. 25 juni 2020 [6/11-2023]. Available from: https://sverigesradio.se/artikel/7502688

245. Olsson, Emma. Läraren [Internet]. FOHM stoppar insamlingen om skolan. 18 januari 2021 [26/12-2021]. Available from: https://www.lararen.se/nyheter/coronaviruset/fohm-stoppar-insamlingen-om-skolan

246. Schau, Oscar; Kerpner, Joachim. Aftonbladet [Internet]. Gymnasieskolor ska gå över till distansundervisning. 17 mars 2020 [4/7-2021]. Available from: https://www.aftonbladet.se/nyheter/a/mR44yl/gymnasieskolor-ska-ga-over-till-distansundervisning

247. Henley, Jon. The Guardian [Internet]. Sweden's Covid-19 strategist under fire over herd immunity emails. 17th August 2020 [16/10-2022]. Available from: https://www.theguardian.com/world/2020/aug/17/swedens-covid-19-strategist-under-fire-over-herd-immunity-emails

7.5.5 Sweden ruining it for other countries

248. Fria Tider [Internet]. Finsk läkare varnar för Sverige: "Alla coronafall kommer därifrån". 26 maj 2020 [26/12-2021]. Available from: https://www.friatider.se/finsk-lakare-varnar-sverige-alla-coronafall-kommer-darifran

249. Begg, Keith; Flyg, Virpi. Worldsocialistwebsite. How Swedish authorities worked to export "herd immunity" to other countries. 5 June 2022 [15/10-2022]. Available from: https://www.wsws.org/en/articles/2022/06/06/swed-j06.html

250. TravelNews.. Här släpper de inte in svenska turister. 12 juni 2020 [26/12-2021]. Available from: https://www.travelnews.se/arrangor/har-slapper-de-inte-in-svenska-turister/

251. McNally, Alan. The Guardian. Backers of 'herd immunity' shouldn't have been allowed near Boris Johnson. 14 December 2020 [7/1-2022]. Available from: https://www.theguardian.com/commentisfree/2020/dec/14/herd-immunity-boris-johnson-coronavirus

7.5.6 Covid healthcare

252. Bergström, Mikael. Region Jönköpings län. 2020. IVA-personal:
Covid-19 kan ge allvarliga symtom som kräver intensivvård.
https://www.rjl.se/nyheter/nyheter-och-pressmeddelanden/iva-personal-
covid-19-kan-ge-allvarliga-symtom-som-kraver-intensivvard-68644 [1/11-
2021]

253. Mossige-Norheim, Thea. 2021. Krav på egen mätning efter Pisa-
skandalen. *Aftonbladet*. 18 maj. https://www.expressen.se/nyheter/krav-pa-
egen-matning-efter-pisa-skandalen/ [17/8-2021]

254. Weilenmann, Leni. 2021. Grönt ljus att rekrytera iva-personal från
Norge och Danmark. *Vårdfokus*. 31 maj.
https://www.vardfokus.se/nyheter/gront-ljus-att-rekrytera-iva-personal-fran-
norge-och-danmark/ [16/10-2022]

255. Älverbrandt, Marcus. 2021. Regioner väntas köpa vård för att klara
köerna. *Aftonbladet*. 9 oktober.
https://live.aftonbladet.se/supernytt/news/regioner-vaentas-koepa-vaard-
foer-att-klara-koeerna.iQZAbKSek [1/11-2021]

256. Angry Foreigner. 2020. *Whistleblower M.D. - Sweden Refusing Oxygen
to Older Patients.* https://www.youtube.com/watch?v=Kz5BhX5_CXo
[10/9-2022]

257. Blavier, Johanna. 2020. Regionen bekräftar rykten om att alla inte får
syrgas. *Sveriges radio*. 22 april. https://sverigesradio.se/artikel/7458165
[6/12-2021]

258. Kadhammar, Peter. 2020. Andningsskydd för alla svenskar brändes upp
– utan protester. *Aftonbladet*. 2 April.
https://www.aftonbladet.se/nyheter/kolumnister/a/BRXn37/andningsskydd-
for-alla-svenskar-brandes-upp--utan-protester [6/12-2021]

259. Petrsson. (2020). *Anders Ygeman: Glöm lager med livsmedel,
skyddsmasker och andra förnödenheter*.
https://petterssonsblogg.se/2020/04/06/anders-ygeman-glom-lager-med-
livsmedel-skyddsmasker-och-andra-fornodenheter/ [22/9-2022]

260. Svensson, Olof. 2020. Larmet från coronavården: Masker och visir slut om två dagar. *Aftonbladet.* 12 december. https://www.aftonbladet.se/nyheter/a/wPjOR4/larmet-fran-coronavarden-masker-och-visir-slut-om-tva-dagar [6/12-2021]

261. Nilsson, Johannes. 2020. Svenonius om bristen på skyddsutrustning: "Jag tror ingen såg det komma". *Nyheteridag.* 1 april. https://nyheteridag.se/svenonius-om-bristen-pa-skyddsutrustning-jag-tror-ingen-sag-det-komma/ [22/9-2022]

262. Almgren. 2020. Regnrockar från Gröna Lund blir skyddskläder på Karolinska. *Samnytt.* 19 april. https://samnytt.se/regnrockar-fran-grona-lund-blir-skyddsklader-pa-karolinska/ [6/12-2021]

7.5.7 Prioritisations in the healthcare

263. Svensson, Olof. 2020. Dokument visar: De prioriteras bort från intensivvård. *Aftonbladet*. 9 April. https://www.aftonbladet.se/nyheter/samhalle/a/lAyePy/dokument-visar-de-prioriteras-bort-fran-intensivvard [13/11-2021]

264. Andersson, Sara. 2020. Socialstyrelsen: "Yngre i dåligt skick kan prioriteras bort". *Världen idag*. 20 maj. https://www.varldenidag.se/nyheter/socialstyrelsen-yngre-i-daligt-skick-kan-prioriteras-bort/reptet!Po@lqpKd0623gCMn30WJw/ [13/11-2021]

265. Spencer, Robert. 2018. Sweden's Minister of Social Affairs claims country's elderly, not Muslim migrants, are "the big problem". *JIHAD WATCH*. 30th April. https://www.jihadwatch.org/2018/04/swedens-minister-of-social-affairs-claims-countrys-elderly-not-muslim-migrants-are-the-big-problem [13/11-2021]

266. Fjällsjö nyheter. 2020. *Äldreboende försökte döda coronasjuk pensionär*. https://www.xn--fjllsj-cua2m.se/nyheter/20200521-aldreboende-corona-pensionar [13/11-2021]

267. Salihu, Diamant. 2020. Professorns ilska mot coronavården av äldre: "Är diskriminering". *Svt*. 22 April. https://www.svt.se/nyheter/professorns-ilska-mot-coronavarden-av-aldre-ar-diskriminering [13/11-2021]

268. Karlsson, Josefine. 2020. Eva, 96, nekades coronatest – dottern Catharina såg henne dö på äldreboendet. *Aftonbladet*. 9 April. https://www.aftonbladet.se/nyheter/a/rARez3/eva-96-nekades-coronatest--dottern-catharina-sag-henne-do-pa-aldreb [13/11-2021]

269. Malm, Sara. 2020. Hallåans sorg: Mamman dog i misstänkt corona. *Expressen*. 8 april. https://www.expressen.se/nyheter/coronaviruset/hallaans-sorg-mamman-dog-i-misstankt-corona/ [13/11-2021]

7.5.8 Tegnell on Lockdown

270. Payne, Adam. Buissnesinsider. A new Swedish coronavirus antibody study suggests the herd-immunity strategy isn't working. May 21st 2020 [10/10-2022]. Available from:
https://www.businessinsider.com/coronavirus-antibody-study-suggests-sweden-not-reaching-herd-immunity-2020-5?r=US&IR=T

271. Juhlin, Johan. Svt. Regeringen: Max åtta personer tillåtna vid sammankomster. 17 November 2020 [9/10-2022]. Available from:
https://www.svt.se/nyheter/inrikes/lofven-det-kravs-mer-av-forbud-for-att-fa-ned-kurvan

7.6.1 Vaccine

272. Folkhälsomyndigheten. 2021. *Rekommendationer om prioritetsordning för vaccination mot covid-19.*
https://www.folkhalsomyndigheten.se/smittskydd-beredskap/utbrott/aktuella-utbrott/covid-19/vaccination-mot-covid-19/rekommendationer-for-vaccination-mot-covid-19/ [25/10-2021]

273. Blomberg, Lovisa. 2021. Problem med att folk tränger sig före i vaccinationskön. *Sveriges radio.* 23 februari.
https://sverigesradio.se/artikel/problem-med-att-folk-tranger-sig-fore-i-vaccinationskon [25/10-2021]

274. Riks. 2021. *Kroon (SD): Gör det olagligt att tränga sig före i vaccinkön.* https://www.youtube.com/watch?v=gYCiFIihUAc [25/10-2021]

275. Andersson, Lars; Askersund. 2021. Straffa de som tränger sig före i vaccinkön. *Nerikes Allehanda.* 10 mars. https://www.na.se/2021-03-10/straffa-de-som-tranger-sig-fore-i-vaccinkon [25/10-2021]

276. Turdén, Maria. 2021. Fräcka upptäckten: Tränger sig före i vaccinationskön. *Sveriges radio.* 29 april.
https://sverigesradio.se/artikel/personer-tranger-sig-fore-i-vaccinationskon [25/10-2021]

277. Marteus, Ann-charlotte. 2021. Vaccinmyglande chefer borde inte få en andra dos. *Aftonbladet.* 10 februari. https://www.expressen.se/ledare/ann-charlotte-marteus/vaccinmyglande-chefer-borde-inte-fa-en-andra-dos/ [25/10-2021]

278. Hermansson, Mikael. 2021. Mikael Hermansson: Sverige har inte råd att slänga vaccin. *Borås Tidning.* 2 februari.
https://www.bt.se/ledare/sverige-har-inte-rad-att-slanga-vaccin-c1a0db10/ [25/10-2021]

279. TT. 2021. Kaos när folk tränger sig i vaccinationskön. *Aftonbladet.* 3 mars. https://www.aftonbladet.se/nyheter/a/rgmMya/kaos-nar-folk-tranger-sig-i-vaccinationskon [25/10-2021]

7.6.2 Breaktrough cases and the end of the pandemic
280. Coronaheadsup. 2021. *Israel: 60% of severely ill Covid patients are fully vaccinated.* https://www.coronaheadsup.com/asia/israel-60-of-severely-ill-covid-patients-are-fully-vaccinated/ [29/10-2021]

281. Coronaheadsup. 2021. *UK: 60% of UK Covid-19 hospital cases are double vaccinated.* https://www.coronaheadsup.com/europe/uk-60-of-uk-covid-19-hospital-cases-are-double-vaccinated/ [29/10-2021]

282. Hartmann-Boyce, Jamie. 2021. COVID: the reason cases are rising among the double vaccinated – it's not because vaccines aren't working. *The conversation.* 28th July. https://theconversation.com/covid-the-reason-cases-are-rising-among-the-double-vaccinated-its-not-because-vaccines-arent-working-164797 [29/10-2021]

283. Coronaheadsup. 2021. *Wales: The vaccine breakthrough rate for people over 60 is 96%.* https://www.coronaheadsup.com/coronavirus/wales-the-vaccine-breakthrough-rate-for-people-over-60-is-96/ [29/10-2021]

284. Jeffay, Nathan. 2021. Israeli study claims major drop in vaccine protection; experts don't believe it. *The times of Israel.* 21st July. https://www.timesofisrael.com/israeli-study-claims-major-drop-in-vaccine-protection-experts-dont-believe-it/ [29/10-2021]

285. Johansson, Ingrid. 2021. Larmet: Nu smittas allt fler äldre av covid-19. *Mitt I Södermalm.* 25 september. https://www.pressreader.com/sweden/sodermalmdirekt/20210925/281818581978619 [29/10-2021]

286. 1177 Vårdguiden. 2021. *Vaccination mot covid-19.* https://www.1177.se/sjukdomar--besvar/lungor-och-luftvagar/inflammation-och-infektion-ilungor-och-luftror/om-covid-19--coronavirus/om-vaccin-mot-covid-19/vaccination-mot-covid-19/ [29/10-2021]

287. Krona, Isak. 2021. FHM backar från beslutet att inte testa dubbelvaccinerade med symtom. *Sveriges Radio.* 17 november. https://sverigesradio.se/artikel/fhm-backar-fran-beslutet-att-inte-testa-dubbelvaccinerade?utm_source=headtopics&utm_medium=news&utm_campaign=2021-11-17 [1/1-2021]

288. Skoglund, Karolina. 2021. Här är partierna som är för och emot vaccinpass. *svt.* 7 september. https://www.svt.se/nyheter/har-ar-partierna-for-och-emot-vaccinpass [29/10-2021]

289. Norén, Alexander. 2021. Sverige först ut att testa EU:s coronapass. *svt.* 5 maj. https://www.svt.se/nyheter/inrikes/sverige-forst-ut-att-testa-eu-s-coronapass [29/10-2021]

290. Ahlberg, Mattias. 2021. 81 procent vill ha covidpass på konserter och andra live evenemang. *Finanstid.* 2 september. https://finanstid.se/81-procent-vill-ha-covidpass-pa-konserter-och-andra-live-evenemang/ [1/1-2022]

291. Lagerstedt, Jenny. 2022. Experter: Minst 150 000 svenskar smittas av corona – varje dag. *Svt.* 28 januari. https://www.svt.se/nyheter/inrikes/experter-minst-150-000-svenskar-smittas-av-corona-varje-dag [27/9-2022]

292. Fria Tider. 2022. FHM: Dags för femte dos av vaccin mot covid-19. 27 augusti. https://www.friatider.se/fhm-dags-femte-dos-av-vaccin-mot-covid-19 [27/9-2022]

293. Ellyatt, Holly. 2022. Woman catches Covid twice within 20 days, marking a new record. CNBC. 21st April. https://www.cnbc.com/2022/04/21/woman-caught-covid-twice-in-20-days-marking-a-new-record.html [25/9-2022]

294. TT. 2021. Samhället öppnas upp mer – här är alla lättnader som gäller från och med idag. *Vetlandaposten.* 1 juli. https://app.vetlandaposten.se/2021-07-01/samhallet-oppnas-upp-mer--har-ar-alla-lattnader-som-galler-fran-och-med-idag [29/10-2021]

295. Uppskattat. 2021. KLART: Så ska Sverige öppnas upp igen – steg för steg. 28 maj. https://se.laowl.com/klart-sa-ska-sverige-oppnas-upp-igen-steg-for-steg [29/10-2021]

296. Riks. 2021. Jimmie Åkesson på en "korvresa" i Sverige. https://www.youtube.com/watch?v=DHwXsElFVlM [Online] [29/10-2021]